# The Do's and Don'ts of

# HYPOGLYCEMIA

## AN EVERYDAY GUIDE TO LOW BLOOD SUGAR

### TOO OFTEN MISUNDERSTOOD AND MISDIAGNOSED!

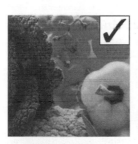

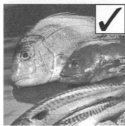
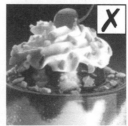

# ROBERTA RUGGIERO

President and Founder of
The Hypoglycemia Support Foundation, Inc.

Frederick Fell Publishers, Inc.
2131 Hollywood Blvd., Suite 305, Hollywood, FL 33020
Phone: (954) 925-5242      Fax: (954) 925-5244
**Web Site: www.FellPub.com**

# Frederick Fell Publishers, Inc.

2131 Hollywood Boulevard, Suite 305

Hollywood, Florida 33020

954-925-5242

**e-mail: fellpub@aol.com**

**Visit our Web site at www.fellpub.com**

This publication is designed to provide accurate and authoritative information in regard to the subject matter covered. It is sold with the understanding that the publisher is not engaged in rendering legal, accounting, or other professional service. If legal advice or other assistance is required, the services of a competent professional person should be sought. From A Declaration of Principles jointly adopted by a Committee of the American Bar Association and a Committee of Publishers.

The information in this book is not intended as medical advice. Its intention is solely informational and educational. It is assumed that the reader will contact a medical or health professional should the need for one be warranted.

## Library of Congress Cataloging-in-Publication Data

Ruggiâero, Roberta, 1942-
  The do's and don'ts of hypoglycemia : an everday guide to low blood sugar / Roberta Ruggiero.
      p. cm.
Previously published: 1988.
  ISBN 0-88391-087-X
1.  Hypoglycemia--Popular works.  I. Title.
  RC662.2.R84 2003
  616.4'66--dc21

                                    2003000277

10 9 8 7 6 5 4 3 2 1
Graphic Design: Elena Solis

# WORDS OF ENDORSEMENT AND PRAISE

"*The Do's and Don'ts of Low Blood Sugar* was chosen among the top best lay medical books because it covers a subject of potential interest to public library patrons in a responsible, easily understood way... A worthwhile edition to a public library collection."

—*American Library Journal*

"*The Do's and Don'ts of Low Blood Sugar* has been endorsed in our programs. Only those books that are felt to be truly outstanding selections are incorporated into our programming. It's always a personal pleasure to encounter and recommend good, conscientious work to our audience."

—*The Midwest Book Review*
Oregon, Wisconsin

"You've done a superb job after years of both personal and intellectual research on this topic. Thank you for helping so many people who will benefit from your experiences and clear writing."

—*Jeffrey S. Bland, Ph.D.*
Gig Harbor, Washington

"This is a great book. So easy and so practical. Just right for the hypoglycemic who seems to fade after concentrating for 10 minutes. You are writing for all those with a short attention span."

—*Lendon H. Smith, M.D.*
Portland, Oregon

"Congratulations on a great book that really brings the whole question of low blood sugar into an easy to read, understandable form. You certainly answer every conceivable question that a patient is likely to ask and I wish you every success."

—*Robert Buist, Ph.D.*
Sydney, Australia

"I appreciate having received your book. The focus for me was the chapter which you discussed the approach to a positive attitude. I love the way you formulated your concepts and am happy for you that the book is in print."

—*Leonard A. Wisneski, M.D., F.A.C.P.*
Bethesda, Maryland

"My first suggestion to a hypoglycemic patient is to read your book. Education and understanding of hypoglycemia, or LBS, is probably the single most important thing that one can do to deal with this condition and your book is a great place to start."

—*Douglas M. Baird, D.O., P.A.*
Tampa, Florida

"Thank you for sending me a copy of your book. The time and effort which you put into it really has paid off. You have an excellent, well written and informative book. I will be sure to show this to my many patients who are suffering with hypoglycemia."

—*Irving Karten, M.D., F.A.C.O.G.*
Hollywood, Florida

"Your latest book on low blood sugar is FANTASTIC! You have successfully distilled the essence of the subject for those that suffer from the often misdiagnosed and misunderstood condition of hypoglycemia. The information on diet, vitamins and exercise could easily be followed by anyone who is seeking health or wants to maintain their health."

—Leo B. Stouder, B.S., D.C., D.N.B.C.E.
Hollywood, Florida.

"As I began to read your book, I couldn't help but feel that I was reading my own story with all the frustrations and fears that you experienced. I would also like to say thanks for all your time and effort you put forth in getting this book published and The Hypoglycemia Foundation started."

—*Madison, Wisconsin*

"The book was a tremendous lift to my spirits and renewed my courage to keep up the pace on the road to recovery. I wish that every person who has hypoglycemia or is suffering the symptoms and doesn't know the cause could read this book. It is a great support!"

—*Selma, North Carolina*

"I believe your book, *The Do's and Don'ts of Low Blood Sugar*, could be the most helpful thing a newly diagnosed hypoglycemic could read. Its simplicity of style makes it an excellent first choice. How I wish it had been available to me in 1980."

—*Del City, Oklahoma*

"I have just finished reading your book, *The Do's and Don'ts of Low Blood Sugar*, which I picked up at the library. It is the most informative book I have found to date."

*—East Lyme, Connecticut*

"My doctor has informed me that I am 'borderline diabetic' and he has recommended that I read the book entitled, *The Do's and Don'ts of Low Blood Sugar*.

*—Summerland Key, Florida*

"...I have scoured bookstores and health food stores and every place else I could think of for information. I was quite discouraged until yesterday when I went to the library. I found a copy of your *Do's and Don'ts of Low Blood Sugar*. I was thrilled with all of the information you included in this book. From my own experience I know how much work must have been involved in gathering it. I finally feel like my husband and I will be able to get a handle on our situation and keep his condition in check."

*—Houston, Texas*

"Your book *The Do's and Don'ts of Low Blood Sugar* was a life saver. After more than 15 years I have finally found my cure: a simple diet!"

*—Poland, Ohio*

"I have read it and found it very helpful. The way it is written makes it very readable and clear and very interesting because it is written from a personal point of view."

*—Southport, Merseyside (England)*

"I read your book recently, *The Do's and Don'ts of Low Blood Sugar.* I wish I had found it before I did all my technical reading. The book made me cry. It also made me feel as if I was being hugged and comforted by a dear friend. You wrote so well about all the things I've been trying to explain to my family as well as to my doctor."

—*Kew Garden Hills, New York*

"I want to thank you for opening up a new world for me."

—*Ft. Lauderdale, Florida*

"It was like looking in a mirror to read your book."

—*Ft. Lauderdale, Florida*

"Since I read your book—it has saved my life-literally."

—*Paris, Kentucky*

"I am a 38 year-old hypoglycemic, recently diagnosed and I cannot thank you enough, Roberta Ruggiero. It was because of your book—*The Do's and Don'ts of Low Blood Sugar,* that I was able to recognize myself as a hypoglycemic, and I asked my doctor to test me. He, although skeptical, agreed, and to my delight my hypoglycemia was confirmed beyond a doubt. This singular diagnosis has finally explained a lifetime of symptoms, physical and emotional, and has helped me and those nearest to me understand that it was not nor is not my "nature" to be miserable, touchy, disagreeable, negative, etc, etc, but it is only a very controllable disorder which causes me to become that way."

—*Niagara Falls, New York*

"Thank you for changing my life!"

—*Holland, Michigan*

"I thank you once again on behalf of our patrons, and we look forward to utilizing your reference materials and to making good use of your help, and guidance in order to improve the care and services we provide to our community!"

May God bless you!
Thanking you for your kindness,

—*Dr. A.N. Malpani, M.D.*
Medical Director
Bombay, India

"I am a Health Educator with the Bermuda Diabetes Association. In the last few months there has been an increase in calls from people inquiring about hypoglycemia, and nearly all of them have expressed dissatisfaction with the explanation/advice they received regarding their condition." I found your website via the Alta Vista search engine. I will recommend your book to all future callers to our Association.

Thank you!

—*Jacqui Neath-Myrie*
Diabetes Prevention Programmer Coordinator
Bermuda Diabetes Association

Dedicated . . .


To every hypoglycemic—particularly those who
have been mistakenly told that their symptoms were
"all in their head."

# TABLE OF CONTENTS

The order or length of each topic does not reflect its importance or value.

Table of Contents

**Please Note:** The terms hypoglycemia and low blood sugar are used interchangeably throughout the book, but have the same meaning.

# ACKNOWLEDGEMENTS

The best part about writing this book is remembering everyone who played a role in its creation. They not only influenced my work, but my life.

Gratitude goes to all the people who suffer with hypo-glycemia and shared their stories with me as well as every professional, medical or otherwise, who said yes to an interview. Thanks also goes to the Board of Directors, Board of Advisors, and all the members of The Hypoglycemia Support Foundation, Inc. (HSF), as well as to the volunteers who gave so generously of themselves.

I would like to especially recognize the following people: Douglas M. Baird, D.O., Lorna Walker, Ph.D., Hewitt Bruce, Ph.D., Stephen J. Schoenthaler, Ph.D., Shirley S. Lorenzani, Ph.D. and the late Dr. Emanuel Cheraskin, M.D., D.M.D. Each and every one of you was instrumental to my growth. As mentors, teachers, healers, and most of all friends, your directions, reassurances, and confidences gave me the courage to continue working toward my dreams.

I would like to give special thanks to: Toni Crabtree, Marie Provenzano, Kimberly Perraud, Karen McCoy, Susan Connors, Carolyn Stein, Tomey Sellars and Dr. Phyllis Schiffer-Simon. On a professional, personal, and spiritual level, each of you combined your strength and support to spur me on during my most difficult times.

Acknowledgements

Special thanks go to the late Harvey M. Ross, M.D. for writing the preface; to David Kohn, Melodee Putt, and Candace Hoffmann for using their editing expertise to polish this manuscript; and to my son-in-law, Charles Stewart, D.M.D. for his valuable suggestions. My deepest gratitude goes to Don Lessne, my publisher; Elena Solis, Graphic Designer; and Lori Sindell Horton, Production Manager/Editor at Frederick Fell Publishers. Each one of you gave my book extra love and tender care from the moment it was placed in your hands.

To my children, Renee and Anthony, and my husband, Tony—your unconditional love, patience, and understanding, gave me the freedom to do my work and to make this book a reality. I am forever grateful.

To my grandchildren Krystina, Cody, Sara, and Stephen— you have made me see the world through your eyes. What more could I ask for?

Last, but definitely not least, my deepest appreciation goes to Theresa Mantovani without whom this book would not have been possible. I miss you dearly.

# PREFACE

I have treated people with hypoglycemia since the late 1960s. I've learned by listening to my patients about the multiple frustrations that they experience, starting from the time they first begin to recognize something is wrong to the numerous visits to doctors over the years. Then, too, there are the frustrations experienced in their professional and personal lives right through to the confusion in treatments and difficulty in adhering to a program once it is outlined. Through her experience, first as a patient, then as an advisor who reaches out to thousands of others to help them through their difficult times, Roberta Ruggiero has learned to help people recognize this illness, find professional help and, finally, help to comply with the programs suggested for the treatment of hypoglycemia.

In *The Do's and Don'ts of Low Blood Sugar*, Roberta shares with her readers the rich knowledge of her own experience. She is able to guide, teach and support those with this problem; a problem that is, more often than not, overlooked or even scoffed at by the majority of those in the medical profession.

If you have, or even suspect that you or someone you know has hypoglycemia, this is the book for you. By following the "do's and don'ts," those with hypoglycemia will be able to reduce and even eliminate their symptoms, and start on the road to a more fulfilling life.

*—Harvey M. Ross, M.D.*
Los Angeles, California

# THE DO'S AND DON'T OF HYPOGLYCEMIA: AN EVERYDAY GUIDE TO LOW BLOOD SUGAR
## Introduction to the Third Edition

The first edition of *The Do's and Don'ts of Low Blood Sugar: An Everyday Guide To Hypoglycemia* was written in 1988 with a tremendous amount of fear and self-doubt. I was writing a medical book with no medical degree and writing about a condition the medical community labeled a non-disease. Even those who recognized its existence, still called hypoglycemia the most confusing, complicated, misunderstood, and misdiagnosed condition of the 21st century.

So, why did I write it in the first place? Why a second revision in 1993? And more importantly, why am I back again in 2003, writing another updated edition? It is because of YOU, my readers. You have written to me, cried on my shoulder, begged for more answers, more information and more research.

From big cities such as Los Angeles, California to little-known towns such as Soddy, Tennessee; from Canada to Great Britain; from Alaska to Ireland, the letters pour in. And since The Hypoglycemia Support Foundation, Inc. launched its website, www.hypoglycemia.org, in 1997; e-mails arrive on a daily basis from around the world. I correspond with hypoglycemics in China, India, Africa, Pakistan, and the Kingdom of Bahrain right from my office in Sunrise, Florida. How incredible, God's plan!

Because 99 percent of those writing to me ask questions concerning hypoglycemia, I strongly believe that the word hypoglycemia should get top billing. No matter what we call it, whether low blood sugar or a blood sugar management disorder, hypoglycemia is the term most of you recognize. Thus, this edition will be called *The Do's and Don'ts of Hypoglycemia: An Everyday Guide to Low Blood Sugar.*

This book includes four new chapters. Three of them address areas of significant concern: hypoglycemia and children, hypoglycemia and alcoholism, and hypoglycemia and diabetes. Although I touch briefly on these topics in this edition, please realize that they all merit further attention and investigation. The fourth chapter provides answers to the most commonly asked questions about hypoglycemia.

Once again, the teachers, advisors, and mentors who assisted me, and The Hypoglycemia Support Foundation, Inc. for the past 22 years, have given their time and expertise to this updated edition. Their dedication and commitment have enabled the HSF to continue, to succeed, and to grow beyond our wildest expectations.

However, despite all of their support, and even though I know that this is my mission, I must admit, there have been times when I've wanted to give up. My strength, determination, and persistence would waver. I would say, "That's it! No more, I quit!" And then someone would call or write and say..."Wow, your book saved my life,"... or..."Your information saved my marriage,"... or..."I thought I was alone but now I feel as though I have an understanding friend."

Sometimes I feel very selfish. I can't tell you what these letters and phone calls mean to me. In helping others, I believe I'm really helping myself. I've grown emotionally, intellectually, mentally, and spiritually. I think that's what life is all about—living life to its fullest.

I have been blessed a hundred fold. The people I have met, been privileged to work with, share with, confide in, laugh and cry with—my family, friends, brothers, and sisters of this incredible universe—you are among my greatest blessings.

# INTRODUCTION

If you think you may be going crazy; if you have thoughts of suicide; if you're constantly exhausted, anxious and depressed; if you go for weeks without a decent night's sleep; if your personality changes like the flip of a coin; if a counter full of munchies doesn't satisfy your sweet tooth; and if your doctor thinks you must be a hypochondriac because medical tests don't show anything physically wrong with you—don't despair, there's hope!

You may not need a psychiatrist, or even pain pills, tranquilizers or anti-depressants. Surprisingly, a simple DIET may relieve your symptoms!

This condition, which is confusing, complicated, misunderstood and too often misdiagnosed, is hypoglycemia, or low blood sugar. According to leading medical authorities, it affects one-half of all Americans, including celebrities Burt Reynolds and Merv Griffin. It is most frightening because most people who have it, don't know it. Often, the myriad collection of symptoms are blamed on other causes.

I know because I've been there. I suffered with hypoglycemia for ten years. Numerous medical specialists, dozens of tests, thousands of pills, and even the administration of electroconvulsive shock therapy (ECT), did nothing to eliminate my symptoms.

A simple glucose tolerance test (GTT), proper diet and strong determination finally led me down the road to recovery. Unfortunately, it took years. If only I had had the knowledge that lies between the covers of this book, my journey would not have been so traumatic.

To help others avoid what I experienced, to bring to them the causes and effects of hypoglycemia, and to give support, encouragement and enlightenment to those suffering this insidious disease, I formed The Hypoglycemia Support Foundation Inc. (HSF) on June 6, 1980.

Through the HSF, I have had the opportunity to speak with thousands of "searching" hypoglycemics. They all are looking for the best doctor, diet, book or miracle cure. They are asking the questions that I once asked: What should I eat? Should I take vitamins? Should I exercise? Why isn't my diet working? Why doesn't my family understand? Can I ever eat out again? More serious questions commonly asked are:Why doesn't my doctor recognize hypoglycemia? He says it's just a "fad" disease. Is the glucose tolerance test necessary? How can I find a physician sympathetic to a hypoglycemic's needs? The list is endless, and so, sometimes, is the pain.

During this time, as I was trying to educate hypo-glycemics, they in turn, educated me. They told me what they needed and wanted and, above all, what they were not getting. I learned of their pitfalls, anxieties and fears. Coupled with my own feelings, everyone I encountered seemed to respond with the same universal phrase, "If only I had known . . ."

There are many good books out on the subject of hypoglycemia. However, when I insisted that a patient get a book to read about his or her condition, I began to realize that most of the people were in the first stages of hypoglycemia, a time when the mind is confused, the body is weak and concentration is difficult.

When I found myself repeating the same guidelines over and over again, I realized that these patients first needed simple, concise and comprehensible guidelines to help them handle their condition. They needed a prerequisite, a book to read BEFORE all the other books on hypoglycemia. They needed a book with specific do's and don'ts written in layperson's vocabulary before grasping for medical definitions and explanations.

This is what I hope to achieve with *The Do's and Don'ts of Hypoglycemia*. Use it as a key to education, interweave it with commitment and then, love yourself enough to take the final step—application! Are you ready?

"To be sugar free in a sugar coated
world is a nightmare!"

Donna 1990

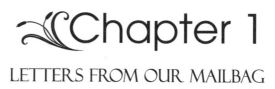

# Chapter 1

## LETTERS FROM OUR MAILBAG

Why devote a chapter strictly to letters and e-mails that I have received? The answer is quite simple. I am hoping the following correspondence will have the same effect on you as it had on me. I am hoping that the connection that was formed, the bond that was cemented and the feeling that flowed between the writer and me will be passed on to you, my reader. I want you to benefit by gaining inspiration from the challenges and triumphs experienced by other hypoglycemics and learn from their mistakes and their successes.

Together, let's shed more light on hypoglycemia which it needs if the sting is to removed from it's tail. The following letters will speak for themselves.

Dear Roberta:

THANK YOU, THANK YOU, THANK YOU!
The information you have been kind enough to share with me has been the key link enabling me to return to a normal life.

Several months ago, I began growing faint and was, on about half a dozen occasions, taken to the emergency room of a local hospital.  In every instance, I was told there was nothing wrong and that I was probably just hyperventilating. After consulting several doctors without any success at all, I was properly diagnosed by a local physician who recommended a glucose tolerance test.  Once it was determined that I had hypoglycemia, I was referred to the Cleveland Clinic for dietary planning.

The staff at the Cleveland Clinic were enormously helpful but referred me to you and your organization for additional help. The materials you have supplied me have helped me understand my problem and do what is necessary to return to a normal life.  I am saddened by my own experience with the many doctors who were unable to determine what was wrong with me.  I am frightened for the many thousands of patients throughout the country with similar problems who are no doubt experiencing the same kind of difficulty with their diagnosis.  I hope for their sake that they will be as fortunate as I was to be directed to you and your wonderful, caring organization.

Please let me know if there is anything I can ever do to repay the enormous debt I owe to you.

Sincerely,
Fort Lauderdale, Florida

Dear Roberta,

Thank you...Since I read your book (it saved my life, literally) about three years ago, I've been on again, and off again the diet. I usually go back on my diet after a very bad episode, such as my pancreas killing me, or I start blacking out again.

Only those who have had this devastating illness can understand how one understanding person who writes a book (you & your book) can save so many people from unnecessary reactions such as suicide.

I wrote to you once before several years ago crying my eyeballs out. Finally, after my entire life and several doctors telling me everything but, hypoglycemia, it was good to know I was not nuts.

Thank You!
Paris, Kentucky

Dear Roberta,

I have just finished reading your wonderful book for the second time and I can't tell you how much it helped me. It's such a terrible disease to have, it was the most trying time of my whole life, I thought I was going insane for sure. It started out for me about seven months ago, I got out of bed one morning and started to have a panic attack, (which I had never experienced one in my life), and thought I was having a heart attack. My husband was at work and my children, ages seven and three, were still asleep, so I called my neighbor and she took me to the hospital. They told me it was my nerves, gave me a shot and sent me home. After that I kept having panic attacks, anxiety, and severe depression. I went to my doctor and he gave me nerve pills and said that it had to be something in my subconscious that was triggering all of my symptoms. I just knew that it was something physical because I started to develop a lot of other symptoms after that. I would go back to my doctor and tell him that the pills weren't helping, about the other symptoms I was getting and he almost acted mad because I wouldn't take his word for it. I feel that God really had his hand in all of this because my family and friends were all praying for me and my neighbor (who took me to the hospital), her daughter has hypoglycemia and she thought that I could have it, because she had the same symptoms that I was having. So, I went back to my doctor again and I asked him if he thought I could have low blood sugar. He sort of laughed and said that most people who have panic attacks think they have that or else a brain tumor.

I feel that he just agreed to give me a five hour GTT to humor me, I think it really offended him because I was

right and he was wrong.  My blood sugar level went down
to 46 in the third hour of my test, when I called his office
to get the results, he didn't even talk to me on the phone,
his receptionist told me I had low blood sugar and made an
appointment for me to see a dietician at the hospital.  She,
(the dietician), was very helpful and she even said she
couldn't understand why doctors don't recognize and
check people for hypoglycemia more often. Three days later
I called a different doctor and made an appointment and
had all of my medical records transferred over to him. Well,
I am so happy that I switched doctors. My new doctor took
a complete family history and said that I am a prime candi-
date for hypoglycemia with having diabetes in my family,
and I also had diabetes with my first pregnancy. He felt that
46 on my GTT was no doubt low and he's following up on
everything, too. He wants to see me every six months to
check for diabetes and to see how I am doing.

I am so thankful that I didn't have to suffer a real long
time, like you or some of the other poor people in your
book, before I found out what was wrong. I am thankful
that I now have a lot more good days than bad ones.  It is
so nice to have a doctor who is understanding and recog-
nizes how dreadful it is to have this disease. I just don't
understand why all doctors don't recognize hypoglycemia.
It is really a shame to think that there are so many people
out there who are having terrible mental and physical problems, and they probably have low blood sugar, I might

never know that they can feel better just by following a diet!

Thank you for writing your book and sharing your story with so many others, I'm sure it has been very helpful to everyone who reads it, and thank you for forming the HSF.

Thank-you
Saginaw, Michigan

Dear Ms. Ruggiero:

I recently came across your book *The Do's and Don'ts of Low Blood Sugar* and would very much appreciate any information (nutritional or otherwise) you may have regarding hypoglycemia. As I began to read your book, I couldn't help but feel that I was reading my own story with all the frustrations and fears that you experienced. I would also like to say thanks for all your time and effort you put forth in getting this book published and The Hypoglycemia Foundation started.

After 10 years of being treated as a manic depressive, 20 electroconvulsive shock therapy (ECT) treatments, and being placed on every anti-psychotic and anti-depressant medication on the market, I was finally diagnosed as hypoglycemic. Since I have changed my diet accordingly, I feel

100% better the majority of the time.

Thank you for your time and attention you have given this letter. I have suffered quite extensively these last 15 years and have no desire to repeat this experience! Therefore, any information that you can provide me with will be most helpful.

Sincerely,
Madison, Wisconsin

Mrs. Ruggiero,

I was so happy to have found your book, *The Do's and Don'ts of Low Blood Sugar.* I'm 26 and have known for several years that I had hypoglycemia but knew little more than to stop eating sugar. I followed the "sacred diet" faithfully for years but never seemed to get much better. When I asked about what to do I was given another copy of that diet, patted on the back and  was told that I would be just fine if I left the sugar alone. When I called the office confused and wilted, I was told to get a candy bar and that would bring my sugar up and I would be fine. The confusion mounted. That was when I decided I would find out on my own what I should do.  So, I hit the libraries, and that is where I found your book.  I felt like you had written the book after spending a few months watching me. It really was nice to finally know that I was dealing with something conquerable.

Your book marks the beginning of my quest for information on this quiet culprit, who sets up camp in the corner of your life, and robs you of your senses. Even though I still find myself in unexplainable tears or wrapped in a blanket in 90 degree weather, I finally feel hope. I feel sure that God has His hand in this matter. Thank you for writing and sharing your experiences and knowledge.

God Bless You,
Milford, Michigan

Dear Mrs. Ruggiero,

I can't tell you how enlightening your book, *Do's & Don'ts of Low Blood Sugar*, was for me. My daughter was diagnosed with hypoglycemia in August of '91.We had been having problems with our daughter since around puberty, she is now 17. Her grades were slipping, she was always in a strange mood and her temper seemed to flash out of the blue. She just didn't seem like a happy adolescent. My daughter has always been independent and a handful but I thought these changes were just part of puberty.

When we would get on her about school she would tell us she was studying but found it hard to remember what she read. My husband and I would just shake our heads and say she just wasn't putting enough effort into her work. We even had her tested for LD problems but the test proved negative. By the time she entered high school she was having headaches, first thing in the morning, which I figured could be a migraine but she never liked school, was doing poorly, so I figured most times it was a ruse to get out of school. Then we started with dizziness and she was complaining of almost passing out. At this point we took her to the doctor. She had the Glucose Tolerance Test (over 5 hours) and was diagnosed. We were given a diet, told this was common in teens and she would probably outgrow the problem. It seemed no big deal. The doctor said to keep her on the diet for three months then start reintroducing foods—looking for the dizziness as a guide. Artificial sweeteners were fine, and natural fruit juices were also acceptable, no restricted amounts.

By this time I had talked my husband into family counseling. It seemed what I thought was a family was disintegrating around me. I was an emotional mess. It never dawned on me to read up on her hypoglycemia. I could only concentrate on one thing at a time and counseling was it.

Counseling seemed to be helping out but we still had periods of uneven behavior. I had read an article in the paper about behavior problems with hypoglycemic kids and asked the doctor if this was   true. He said, "No way, don't give her that handle to use." I believed him.  Why?  I can't answer that, not even now. After a year almost, all of the foods had been reintroduced. She has reported no dizziness but erratic behavior, even worse than before. Our counselor had her evaluated by a psychiatrist who diagnosed a long term depression. When she was arrested for battery last week I called our counselor and asked for his help. His first thought was a reevaluation.  His supervisor overruled this and they had a staff meeting instead.  In the meeting was the supervisor, our counselor, the psychiatrist and a psychologist. They concluded that she had a "Personality Disorder" and we had to accept her as is and we were on our own and then they wished us good luck.

Two days after this verdict my daughter brought home your book. (My daughter works at a library.) I can't even describe how I felt as I read this book. The pain, the guilt, the unbelief that I could be unaware of this for so long. That I had put my daughter through hell because I didn't do my job as a mother. I tried calling the counselor. I didn't even know if he told the staff that my daughter has hypoglycemia. We had told him when we first started the sessions. He was honest with us.  He told us he knew nothing about it, we explained what we knew from the doctor and promptly forgot about it.

I don't know how to pull this together.  I can't let this diagnosis stand as is if the hypoglycemia wasn't taken into account, which I feel it wasn't. I know that my daughter will not miraculously turn into Mary Poppins but if LBS accounts for even a small percentage of her problems I feel it should be reevaluated.

I need advice. I've set this trap by my own ignorance but I don't want my daughter to pay for my mistakes.

Sincerely,
Mokena, Illinois

Dear Mrs. Ruggiero,

Thank you for writing your book, *The Do's and Don'ts of Low Blood Sugar.*

In 1980 I was diagnosed as hypoglycemic by an alert and caring physician. Bless him! Even though I was not subjected to many of the horrors most hypoglycemics experience when they first realize 'something' is wrong I well remember the feeling of having been transported to some twilight zone where nothing made sense as I struggled to understand my condition. My own experience convinced me it takes two people, a knowledgeable doctor and an informed patient, to manage this condition. In my attempts to understand hypoglycemia, what it is and how to treat it, I read most of the literature available to the average person. Given my belief that education is essential to the hypoglycemic, it is still my policy to read everything available on the subject. I believe your book, *The Do's and Don'ts of Low Blood Sugar*, could be the most helpful thing a newly-diagnosed hypoglycemic could read. Its simplicity of style makes it an excellent first choice. How I wish it had been available to me in 1980.

Sincerely
Del City, Oklahoma

Dear Sirs,

I was thrilled to find Roberta Ruggiero's book, *The Do's and Don't of Low Blood Sugar*, and find out about your organization! My symptoms of hypoglycemia began in 1984 after the birth of my daughter. I knew there was nothing physically wrong with me so I thought I must have been going crazy. My mood changes were too frequent and drastic to be normal. I knew we could not afford a psychiatrist so I made an effort to cope with the problems on my own. It may have been a blessing in disguise, however, because I was not given tranquilizers and other drugs and therapy about which I've heard horror stories. My symptoms grew to include sudden hunger, weakness, dizziness, nervousness, fatigue, confusion, depression, etc. I suffered for four and a half years until finally a sympathetic doctor agreed to give me a glucose tolerance test. It was then that my suspicions were confirmed and I discovered that I was definitely hypoglycemic.

It has been almost a year since my GTT and I am finally beginning to feel that I am making progress. My doctor, sympathetic though he was, gave me the wrong advice about my diet telling me that I needed more sugar. As a result I spent about five months eating the wrong things, and my symptoms got much worse instead of better. A friend recognized what was happening to me and put me on the right track. I am doing much better now, but am still not as well as I would like to be.

That is the reason I was so glad to find Mrs. Ruggiero's book. I was beginning to lose ground and get depressed about my condition again, feeling that it was a never-ending battle. The book was a tremendous lift to my spirits and renewed my courage to keep up the pace on the road to recovery. I wish that every person who has hypoglycemia or is suffering the symptoms and doesn't know the cause could read this book. It is a great support!

Thank you so much for such a helpful book and for letting me share my story with you, though I'm sure you've heard it hundreds of times from others! Thank you for all you are doing to help others with hypoglycemia!

Yours truly,
Selma, North Carolina

Dear Mrs. Ruggiero:

I read your book recently *The Do's and Don'ts of Low Blood Sugar*. I wish I had found it before I did all my technical reading. The book made me cry. It also made me feel as if I was being hugged and comforted by a dear friend. You wrote so well about all the things I've been trying to explain to my family, as well as to my doctor.

Sincerely,
Kew Garden Hills, New York

Dear Roberta,

Thank you so much for your call. I can't tell you how honored I felt. Since I got over the shock that my condition was "nutritional" and not "mental," I always felt that there was something I should be doing so that others would not needlessly have to go through what I went through. You took that step and I hope that I can contribute to help spread the word!

Sincerely,
Topeka, Kansas

Dear Dr. Ruggiero,

"My name is Kate and I am a hypoglycemic. I would like to share my story. I am 18 years old, and I was recently diagnosed with the condition about three months ago. Up until then, the doctors didn't know what was wrong with me. When I was 14, I suffered three concussions (from soccer) and ever since then I've had a non-stop headache. They wrote it off as a post concussive syndrome, but little did they know that it was really all from my low blood sugar. I've had a non-stop headache since November 2, 1997. I had other symptoms that related to the symptoms of hypoglycemia. The doctors put me on every medication you can think of, ranging from anti-depressants to anti-seizure medication. I never saw any change, nothing made the pain stop, only certain things made it worse (stress). Throughout the whole four years I was never depressed though, it was strictly for the use of stopping the headache, which it never did. Hypoglycemia is in my family, but I never knew I had it, until I gave up soda for lent this year, 2002, and when I had a small little piece of candy, my headache tripled. So then I asked my doctor what was wrong and he had no clue, he said I might have an allergy to sugar, and so I asked him how we find out, and then I proceeded with the five-hour glucose testing. It was a real shock when the tests came back positive for hypoglycemia. If I didn't stop the soda, I never would have figured it out.

The doctors always threw medicine at me and never once thought to check my blood. From that day on I started seeing a nutritionist and my health has dramatically changed. For the first time in four and a half years I actually felt like I had hope and that I knew I was going to get better. I've been on an amino acid drink, which has helped me so much, and I'm currently trying to get off my medication. I've seen such a difference, that I wish the doctors would have figured it out back then."

Sincerely,
Kate

# ~（Chapter 2

T here was no turning back. After years of trying to hide my deepest secret, I was now sharing it with what seemed to be the world. Tallahassee's "Capitol News" quoted me verbatim on May 9, 1978: It stated that Roberta Ruggiero, a former shock treatment patient from Cooper City, called the therapy "barbaric" saying she would "rather die than go through electric shock again."

The trail from private mental patient to public notoriety started out rather innocently. After my first child was born in 1961, I went into a deep depression. I couldn't stop crying. I had heard of postpartum depression, but mine was a deluge of tears that had no end. My family physician kept assuring me that my reaction was normal, and that it would go away. When it didn't, he introduced me to my first tranquilizer—Valium.

Then the headaches started. The pain was there in the morning when I woke up, and persisted through my waking hours, and sometimes through the night. The pounding got so intense it felt as though my heart was actually throbbing inside my head. I was then given pills to reduce the pain.

I began having difficulty sleeping at night. Trying to get up in the morning was even more of a task. I became tired and weak. Cooking and cleaning the house, which I had always enjoyed, became a dreaded chore. I began to skip breakfast, hardly eat lunch and just nibble at dinner, if I had the energy to cook.

In 1963, I gave birth to my second child. All of my previous symptoms were compounded by dizzy spells and blurred vision. My nerves, needless to say, were hopelessly frazzled. My hands and feet were constantly cold to the point of feeling frostbitten. Even with medication, my symptoms got progressively worse. My doctor put me in the hospital for a multitude of tests: laboratory, x-rays, spinal taps and electroencephalogram. All the tests came out negative. There was nothing physically wrong with me. I began to think beyond a doubt that I was going crazy. I withdrew into a shell, avoiding contact with my family and friends because I was too embarrassed and ashamed to face them.

It was at this point that my doctor recommended psychotherapy. I spent several months with the first psychiatrist. He thought that perhaps the strain of getting married at an early age (18) and having two children 16 months apart, were the major contributing factors to my illness.

Maybe a "contributing factor," but not THE reason. When the psychiatrist put me on heavy doses of anti-depressants, I went to psychiatrist number two. It was a repeat performance.

My pain and symptoms were being drowned with strong medication. I was given pills to calm me down, pills to help me sleep and pills to relieve pain. That was the order of the day. But since medication and therapy were not enough to relieve the symptoms, much less stabilize them, a third psychiatrist suggested electroconvulsive shock therapy, (ECT) known simply as shock treatments! By this time, I was desperate and would have tried anything. The year was 1969, and in addition to all of my physical and emotional pain, I began to feel guilty about what I was putting my husband through. I agreed to go away and have what I believed was the "cure"—my last hope.

I was wrong. I had not anticipated that my hospital room would have bars on the windows and doors. I didn't know that my clothing, wedding ring and "Miraculous Medal" would be taken away. And even more frightening were the screams, stares and glassy eyes of the patients who had already received treatments. I'll never forget the cot and its leather straps that bound my hands and feet, the electrodes that were put on my temples, and the rubber gag inserted in my mouth. The memories haunt me to this day.

After my first treatment, while I still had some faculties intact, I begged to go home, or at least speak to my husband. If he knew what I was going through, he would stop them. They said no. I had signed the papers for a series of electric shock treatments, and that's what I was going to get.

I had eight treatments in eleven days. The results were horrifying. I am thankful I don't remember all of them. I do remember feeling like I was in a state of limbo. My mind was functioning, but not in coordination with the rest of my body. Despair, shame, guilt and thoughts of suicide remained. Approximately ten months later, I reluctantly agreed to another series of treatments, but this time on an out-patient basis. It was at the end of this series, that I swore I would rather die than ever be subjected to electric shock treatments again. The physical pain was nothing compared to the feelings of isolation, embarrassment and humiliation they caused.

With no solution in sight, we took the advice of our family physician who suggested that a change of scenery or a move to another state might offer some relief. It would be like a fresh start. Therefore, when my husband had an opportunity to move to South Florida, we didn't hesitate.

Our move was exciting. I began to feel a little better. The pain in my head began to go away. Just having the sun shine every day seemed to promise a future where none had existed for so long. Then, suddenly, it happened again. This time, though, a new symptom assailed me. I began having fainting spells. I agreed to go for one last medical consultation. Dr. Arthur Ecoff, an osteopathic physician, examined me, reviewed my records and suggested a glucose tolerance test. I had never had this test before and was skeptical that a diagnosis could be reached. At this point, I would have settled for any diagnosis!

The GTT was taken and I was told I had a severe case of functional hypoglycemia. I was ecstatic! At last, I had a diagnosis, a name and a cure! But, to both my bewilderment and surprise, instead of a bottle of pills, injections or vitamins, I was given a DIET! Good-bye Yankee Doodles, Devil Dogs, hot fudge sundaes and apple pie. Hello chicken, fish, fresh vegetables, whole grains and fruits. I thought, "This is going to be a cinch."

Unfortunately, what I hoped would be an "overnight" remedy turned out to take several years of sorting through a mass of confusing and complicated information. Due to the unfamiliarity with the stages of recuperation, the controversy surrounding its treatment, and non-acceptance from many in the medical community, I found myself with the feeling of being the only person in the world suffering from this baffling disease.

Eventually, success did come, but alleviating my symptoms was a long and slow process. It would have been quicker if only I had understood the importance of individualizing my diet, the necessity for vitamins and exercise, and the role a positive attitude plays in the healing process. Above all, if there were other hypoglycemics to lend support and encouragement, the road back to health would not have been so rocky. Faith, patience, determination and the boundless love of my family were the cornerstones to my recovery.

Consequently, I didn't hesitate for a moment when I came across an article in <u>The Miami Herald</u> appealing to anyone who had experienced devastating effects of electric shock treatments. A committee for patients' rights was lobbying in Tallahassee and, after listening to my story, was eager to have me testify before the state legislature on behalf of mental patients. My hope was to convince the lawmakers to put severe restrictions on the use of ECT and, better yet, give the glucose tolerance test before its administration.

Little did I know that my life would never be the same. My story appeared in newspapers and on radio stations. I was immediately inundated with phone calls and mail from all over the state.

*Letters, like the following, became all too familiar.*

"Please send information. I had undiagnosed hypoglycemia for 23 years, and during that time, I ran the whole gamut—depression, weight gain, weight loss, anxiety, psychiatric therapy and institutionalization—until the proper diagnosis was reached. The glucose tolerance test revealed that I had a blood sugar level of 35! Since that time, I am like a new person. I follow the proper diet, enjoy life and have no apprehension about blacking out without notice."

"I was ecstatic to see your article. My case was diagnosed approximately four months ago by my chiropractor. My internist had written me off as either psychotic or a hypochondriac, or both."

This feedback was the inspiration for my decision to start speaking to both hypoglycemics and members of our community.

When I couldn't handle the flood of letters and phone calls, and when I realized I needed medical and professional guidance, the idea to form a support group became a reality.

And so, the formation of The Hypoglycemia Research Foundation, Inc., became official on June 6, 1980 and renamed The Hypoglycemia Support Foundation, Inc. on December 13, 1991. I am proud to say that I believe that no other organization has accomplished so much with so little.

When I say "little," I refer to practically no money, secretarial services, office equipment, supplies, private phone or office space. How did we survive? Through positive people, positive thoughts, endless hours of hard work, dedication and prayer—plenty of prayers.

For seventeen years, from 1980 to 1997, the HSF held monthly meetings. We had medical or professional speakers share their knowledge of hypoglycemia, whether it was from a medical, nutritional, psychological or holistic point of view. We participated in health fairs and seminars while I personally brought the message about hypoglycemia to local organizations, schools and hospitals.

In 1984, I was proud and honored to be coordinator of a research project studying the correlation between diet and behavior in juvenile delinquents. It was under the direction of Stephen J. Schoenthaler, Ph.D., a professor of criminal justice at California State University, Stanislaus. With the help and guidance of Dr. Douglas M. Baird, Dr. Lorna Walker, and Nutritional Biochemist, Jay Foster, the study was conducted at The Starting Place in Hollywood, Florida. The participants were 35 juvenile delinquents willing to find out if there might be a nutritional and physical cause to their behavior.

We tested them physically, psychologically, nutritionally, and chemically. The results, though not conclusive due to

24

lack of a placebo control group, are published in the book *Nutrition and Brain Function* (Craiger Press, Basle, Switzerland, 1987) Future studies using control groups and other scientific criteria are absolutely necessary in this area.

In 1988, I wrote the first edition of *The Do's and Don'ts of Low Blood Sugar. An Everyday Guide To Hypoglycemia.* It was the core of all that I had learned since finally being diagnosed. I wanted to share it in the hope of sparing other hypoglycemics from the pain and suffering I went through.

In 1993, a revised edition of my book came out with two additional chapters. "Letters From Our Mailbag" was a hit with our readers. Hypoglycemics, sharing their experiences, convinced my readers that they were not alone and there was indeed help at hand.

For the last five years I have kept a low profile with the HSF. I needed time to find out exactly what role my organization should play, and what course of action I must take. During this time of re-assessment, I took a leap of faith and launched the HSF's first website, www.hypoglycemia.org. What a journey it has been. I've seen our visitor numbers climb to almost 300,000 as of this writing, over 5500 have responded to our hypoglycemia/diabetes survey, and e-mails and requests for information have come from 25 countries!

*Take a look at what an impact we are having!*

- We are guiding families of hypoglycemic children in the city of Kuwait.
- We are providing hope to teens afflicted with low blood sugar in Marshall, Missouri.
- We are supplying libraries in India with our books and tapes to aid mothers dealing with the frustration of hypoglycemic babies.
- Businessmen in the Philippines are improving their stamina and focus through the application of our information.
- We are lecturing to medical students, encouraging them to recognize and accept hypoglycemia.

Now, this book is in its third printing with a revised edition and a new title. It was written with the same hope of sparking your enthusiasm and planting the seeds of determination, strength and persistence. You need it all in order to learn every single thing about controlling hypoglycemia before it controls you!

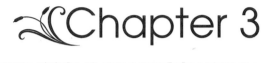

# Chapter 3

## DEFINITIONS OF HYPOGLYCEMIA

I've read and re-read the definition of hypoglycemia at least a hundred times. I've been asked repeatedly, what is hypoglycemia, and, in turn, have asked the leading authorities in the field of preventive and nutritional medicine. Their answers, although similar, are varied. Some are more technical than others. One thing is for certain—the definition of hypoglycemia can be as diversified and complex as the condition itself, or as simple and easy as some of the steps to control it.

In simple layman's language, hypoglycemia is the body's inability to properly handle the large amounts of sugar that the average American consumes today. It's an overload of sugar, alcohol, caffeine, tobacco and stress.

In medical terms, hypoglycemia is defined in relation to its cause. Functional hypoglycemia, the kind we are addressing here, is the over-secretion of insulin by the pancreas in response to a rapid rise in blood sugar or "glucose."

All carbohydrates (vegetables, fruits and grains, as well as simple table sugar), are broken down into simple sugars by the process of digestion. This sugar enters the bloodstream as glucose and our level of blood sugar rises. The pancreas then secretes a hormone known as insulin into the blood in order to bring the glucose down to normal levels.

In hypoglycemia, the pancreas sends out too much insulin and the blood sugar plummets below the level necessary to maintain well-being.

Since all the cells of the body, especially the brain cells, use glucose for fuel, a blood glucose level that is too low starves the cells of needed fuel, causing both physical and emotional symptoms.

*Some of the symptoms of hypoglycemia are:*

*Fatigue, insomnia, mental confusion, nervousness, mood swings, faintness, headaches, depression, phobias, heart palpitations, craving for sweets, cold hands and feet, forgetfulness, dizziness, blurred vision, inner trembling, outbursts of temper, sudden hunger, allergies and crying spells.*

After reading a list like this, one can see why hypoglycemia can be misunderstood and easily misdiagnosed. Don't be alarmed if you read other books that I recommend and see that the list is, in fact, even longer. Don't be confused and frightened when you read other definitions that range from a paragraph to several pages in length.

For the beginner, it is important that you first recognize that most often hypoglycemia is the result of a diet high in sugar, alcohol, caffeine and tobacco.

Before going any further, look at your dietary habits and/or any addictive traits. Start adding up the sodas, coffee, cakes and cigarettes you consume in one day. Keep track of how many meals you miss. Are you under a tremendous amount of stress with your spouse, children, boss, etc. . . ? All of these circumstances can give birth to a case of low blood sugar that can plague you for the rest of your life. Don't take your body for granted. Neglect it, and you'll pay a high price. Take care of it, and low blood sugar becomes an inconvenience that you can manage by yourself.

"Please don't tell me I can never, ever eat a
hot fudge sundae!"

Helena 2001

# ⚔Chapter 4

## IS THERE A DOCTOR OUT THERE?

T he phone rang and I didn't want to answer it. I was going to be late for an appointment 20 minutes away. Reluctantly, I picked up the receiver and a woman's voice said, "Is this The Hypoglycemia Support Foundation?"

"Yes. May I help you?" I asked. She proceeded to tell me her story. It was one that I had heard hundreds of times before, but the tone of her voice was more despondent.

Usually, I can listen attentively, but this time my mind was on my appointment. "Please give me your name and address, and I'll send you some literature."

But the frail voice continued to speak. "Please, please help me. I'm begging you—find me a doctor immediately. I'm anxious and depressed. I can't sleep at night and I can't get up in the morning. I have an incredible craving for sweets. I read an article on hypoglycemia and believe that could be my problem. When I asked my present physician to give me a glucose tolerance test, he refused. He prescribed Valium. Please, before I get hooked on tranquilizers, I want to see a doctor who will listen to me."

I shuddered, and my heart sank. An overwhelming feeling of helplessness set in. I forgot about my appointment and listened to the tortured voice of a person in distress. I wondered to myself, as I had many times before, how many more stories like this one will I have to hear? When will hypoglycemia be accepted as a genuine and serious illness? My own experience and the experience of thousands of others demonstrate that hypoglycemia is real. It does exist. When will the medical profession take it seriously?

In 1980, when I formed the HSF, I wrote to about 50 local physicians looking for help and guidance. I was desperately seeking to arrange places to send the numerous patients who kept asking me where to go for treatment. No one responded. Discouraged and disillusioned, I decided to move beyond my local sphere of influence and contact physicians around the country who knew about hypoglycemia. Astonishingly, a number of them answered.

Emanuel Cheraskin, M.D., D.M.D., Harvey M. Ross, M.D., Jeffrey Bland, Ph.D., E. Marshall Goldberg, M.D.,

Carlton Fredericks, Ph.D. and Robert S. Mendelsohn, M.D., all responded, offering encouragement, support, guidance and hope. Although I was optimistic that I would hear from them, I think deep down inside I was surprised. Probably, because I knew the recent history of hypoglycemia. In the late 1960s and early 1970s, hypoglycemia was written up in a large number of lay publications. The disease suddenly became trendy. It was used as a way to explain some of the worst ills of humanity with little or no scientific backing, and a number of people proclaimed themselves to be hypoglycemics without bothering to consult a doctor or get a glucose tolerance test. The backlash in the medical establishment was swift. In 1949, the American Medical Association (AMA) awarded Dr. Seale Harris its highest honor for the research that led to the discovery of hypoglycemia. After the flood of quackery and self-diagnosis began, the AMA, in 1973, did a 180 degree turn and labeled hypoglycemia a "non-disease."

Don't let this discourage you. There are doctors out there. As the HSF started to gain recognition, acceptance and credibility, doctors from all fields of medicine volunteered their services. From general practitioners in the medical field to osteopaths, chiropractors, nutritionists, and dietitians, they all came. They lectured at our meetings, held seminars, wrote articles and served on our board of directors.

So, don't give up so easily. Take your time, have a positive attitude and follow the HSF's simple guidelines in your search for that special "healer."

**Do**.......... choose a physician carefully but preferably NOT during an emergency situation.

**Do**.......... ask for physician referrals from friends, neighbors, family, business associates, hospitals and organizations.

**Do**.......... read the chapter in this book on the glucose tolerance test, then call the office of someone you are considering and ask the following questions:

a. Do you treat hypoglycemia?

b. How do you test for it?

c. If you administer the glucose tolerance test, how long does it take and how much does it cost?

d. Do you provide nutritional counseling?

e. What is your consultation fee?

f. Are you available by phone if I need to reach you?

g. Will you have time to answer any questions I may have?

h. If I am having financial problems, will you take payments or will you accept my insurance? (ask only if applicable)

**Do**.......... have someone go with you on your first visit. Sometimes, the first visit is an emotional one and you may be nervous or apprehensive. Consequently, questions and/or answers may be misinterpreted or misunderstood. Having a second party along usually helps.

**Do**.......... bring a written list of symptoms, past medical records and personal recollections relating to your present problems. The importance of your past history and the sequence of events leading up to your present condition, cannot be overemphasized.

**Do**.......... bring in a diet/symptom diary (example in back of book). It should include a list of everything you have eaten, including any medication you may have taken in the previous five to seven days. Try to list the time eaten and any symptoms or reactions following consumption. This is important and can be a useful tool for the physician in diagnosing hypoglycemia. However, if you are physically and emotionally unable to do it, DO NOT PANIC—a diagnosis can still be made without it.

**Do**.......... bring in your list of questions. Ask them one at a time and make sure you understand the answer before going on to the next.

35

**Do**.......... tell the physician about any medication you
may be taking at the time. Certain medications
cannot be tolerated by hypoglycemics.

**Do**.......... write down instructions of any kind, or take
along a tape recorder.

**Do**.......... discuss in detail your feelings or concerns, not
just your symptoms. If you have fears you are
not expressing, your treatment will be longer,
more difficult and far more expensive.

**Do**.......... be specific and to the point. The more prepared
you are, the better equipped the doctor will be
to make a proper diagnosis.

**Do**.......... find out if your physician is associated with a
hospital in case of an emergency.

**Do**.......... discuss costs and insurance information. Insurance
companies differ on their policies and willingness
to pay for various tests and procedures. Is your
doctor willing to work out a payment arrangement
and/or accept whatever the insurance company pays?

**Do**.......... get a second opinion, especially if you are not
completely satisfied with the first physician.

**Do**.......... check the office procedures and staff. Do they overbook? Are they friendly? Are they helpful? The last thing you need is a doctor too busy to listen or makes you feel uncomfortable.

**Do**.......... choose a competent, caring, and trustworthy physician who respects your individuality. The doctor-patient relationship is crucial. If your doctor doesn't have your complete confidence or isn't meeting your special needs, then it's definitely time to change.

**Do**.......... notify the physician's office, preferably in writing, if you are upset with the conduct or services of either the physician or the staff.

**Do**.......... discuss a complete prevention program. You need to know how to avoid future health problems, not just how to eliminate the ones you now have. Your current problems are not the only issues that need to be addressed.

**Do**.......... be leery of alternative or new treatment that promises or claims to be a cure-all.

**Do**.......... carry a Health Emergency Card if you're experiencing many LBS symptoms; especially if you've recently blacked-out or fainted. You can

keep your card in your purse, car or briefcase —
any place that can be seen in case of emergency.
To order a Health Emergency Card, please
check the back of the book for details.

**Don't......** call your physician after listening or reading
an article on hypoglycemia and DEMAND a
glucose tolerance test. Instead, take this information, and a list of your symptoms and the
reasons why you feel the test is necessary.
Make an appointment to see your physician
and present him with all the information. If he
appears inattentive or cannot give you a seemingly
justifiable reason why you should not have the
test, look for another physician.

**Don't......** stay with a physician you cannot communicate
with or feel confident about. It will only complicate
existing problems.

**Don't......** call your physician unnecessarily. If your questions
can wait, write them down and save them for
the next visit. The physician will likely have
more time then to give you a better explanation.

**Don't......** wait to call your physician if you're in pain, your symptoms are persistent, or last several days.

**Don't......** continue to be a patient of any physician who just listens for a few minutes and says your symptoms "are all in your head." If you are given a prescription for Valium, get a second opinion as soon as possible.

**Don't......** withhold any medical history out of fear or embarrassment. It is necessary for a proper diagnosis.

**Don't......** seek the advice of a physician and then not follow the instructions issued to you. It's a waste of time and money.

**Don't......** run from one doctor to another. Give each one at least two to four visits to help you.

**Don't......** avoid going to a physician. If your symptoms persist after you've put yourself on a hypoglycemic diet, seek medical advice.

**Don't......** avoid a physician because you lack insurance or money. Ask a family member or friend for financial assistance. You can't afford not to. If it is hypoglycemia, the faster you are diagnosed and treated, the sooner you'll recover.

**Don't**...... demand to be unnecessarily hospitalized.

**Don't**...... hesitate to speak up—ask questions. If you're too timid or embarrassed to communicate with your doctor, then he/she won't be able to adequately meet your needs.

**Don't**...... compare your program or progress with someone else's. Each person's emotional, physical and spiritual make up is unique. A competent physician will tailor a program to fit your individual needs.

**Don't**...... forget, there ARE many caring, sensitive, trustworthy physicians out there. If at first you don't succeed in finding one—try, try again!

# ⁓⁓Chapter 5

## THE IMPORTANCE OF INDIVIDUALIZING YOUR DIET

One of the HSF members called to tell me she was feeling terrible, particularly after eating breakfast. She started to shake, her stomach was nauseous and she felt jittery throughout the morning. She didn't understand why her symptoms were getting worse even though she was staying on a strict diet—no sugar, white flour, caffeine, alcohol or tobacco.

I suggested that we go over her diet but she emphatically said, "It can't be my diet. I eat only what my doctor told me to eat and what the books I read suggested." However, upon my insistence, she started to give me an account of her daily intake of food. First thing every morning, she drank an eight-ounce glass of orange juice. Even though the book she read said to take four ounces, she figured eight should be twice as good.

I didn't let her continue any further. From my own personal experiences, there is no way I can handle orange juice on an empty stomach first thing in the morning. An 8-ounce glass of orange juice, although it is "natural," contains six teaspoons of sugar. For me and many hypoglycemics that I have spoken to, orange juice causes the same reaction as a strong cup of black coffee. The results are the shakes, butterflies in the stomach and an overall feeling of wanting to "jump out of your skin."

At first, it was difficult for this hypoglycemic to understand that if she had this "nervous attack" every morning after eating the same breakfast she should begin to question her diet; not continue to abide by it when she suffered adverse symptoms. We are individuals and thus must tailor every diet to our own bodies when a given diet proves troublesome.

As I mentioned before, there are many books on hypoglycemia. If you've read some of them, by now you're aware that many disagree on what type of diet to follow. It's indeed confusing if you read one book and it tells you to eat a high protein/low carbohydrate diet, while another book says to consume low protein/high carbohydrate foods. Where does that leave you, the confused and bewildered hypoglycemic?

First of all, I am sure that each author has enough confirmation and evidence that his or her diet is successful. Most likely, they all are. Probably, this is due to the fact that the big offenders (sugar, white flour, alcohol, caffeine and tobacco) are eliminated and six small meals are consumed instead.

But the key to a successful diet lies in its "individualization." Each one of us is different. Each one of us is biochemically unique. Therefore, every diet must be tailor-made to meet our individual nutritional requirements.

The list of foods your physician gives you or the list you may read in your favorite book on hypoglycemia, even the suggested food list in the back of this book, are basic guidelines. **Variations come with time and patience, trial and error.** Don't be afraid to listen to your body. It will send you signals when it cannot tolerate a food.

So, basically stick to the suggestions in the following do's and don'ts, and hopefully, with just a few adjustments during your course of treatment, a new and healthier you will gradually appear.

**Do..........** Do keep a daily account of everything you eat for one week to ten days. In one column, list every bit of food, drink and medication that you take and at what time. In the second column, list your symptoms and the time at which you

experience them. Very often you will see a correlation between what you have consumed and
your symptoms. When you do, eliminate those
foods or drinks that you notice are contributing
to your behavior and note the difference. DO
NOT STOP MEDICATION. If you believe that
your medication may be contributing to your
symptoms, contact your physician. A diet diary is
your personal blueprint: a clear overall view of
what you are eating, digesting and assimilating.
It can be the first indicator that something is
wrong and, perhaps, a very inexpensive way of
correcting a very simple problem.

**Do**.......... start eliminating the "biggies"—those foods,
drinks and chemicals that cause the most problems:
sugar, white flour, alcohol, caffeine and tobacco.

**Do**.......... be extremely careful when and how you eliminate the offending substances. Only YOU, with
the guidance of a health care professional, can
decide. Some patients choose to go at a steady
pace. If you drink ten cups of coffee a day, gradually reduce consumption over a period of days
or weeks. The same is true for food or tobacco.
If you are heavily addicted to all of the aforementioned, particularly alcohol, then withdrawal

should not be undertaken unless you are under the care of a physician.

**Do...........** replace offending foods immediately with good, wholesome, nutritious food and snacks as close to their natural state as possible. Lean meats, poultry (without the skin), whole grains, vegetables and allowable fruits are recommended. We want to prevent deprivation from setting in, especially the "poor me, I have nothing to eat" attitude. There is plenty to eat.

**Do..........** eat six small meals a day or three meals with snacks in between. Remember not to overeat.

**Do..........** drink plenty of water. Most physicians say eight glasses of water a day is best.

**Do..........** be aware that when you start on a hypoglycemic diet, you might experience migrating aches, pain in your muscles and/or joints, headaches or extreme fatigue. This is normal when eliminating refined foods. Call your physician if they persist.

**Do..........** be prepared to keep your blood sugar stabilized at all times, whether at home, office, school or traveling. At home you should always have allowable foods ready in the refrigerator or cupboards. Always keep snacks in your car or where you work.

**Do**.......... package food in Tupperware or air-tight containers. Aladdin's insulated thermos jar is handy for cold food and snacks. Aladdin also sells wide-mouth insulated bottles for hot foods, like soups or cut up meat and vegetables. Packaged nuts, seeds, and cheese can be easily carried or stored in a purse or in jacket pockets. You can buy almost everything you need at a supermarket.

**Do**.......... rotate your foods. Eating the same foods over and over again for consecutive days can result in food sensitivities or allergies.

**Do**.......... read labels. Avoid ALL sugars—dextrose, fructose, glucose, lactose, maltose and sucrose. Read labels in health food stores too. Just because you buy something in a health food store, does not necessarily mean you can tolerate the ingredients.

**Do**.......... avoid artificial sweeteners, additives, preservatives and food coloring. Monosodium Glutomate

(MSG) is a big problem for many hypoglycemics —avoid it completely.

**Do**.......... watch your fruit consumption. If you are in the early or severe stage of hypoglycemia, you may not be able to eat any fruit. Some patients can eat just a small amount. Your diet diary will help guide you. Avoid dried fruits completely.

**Do**.......... be careful of the amount of "natural" foods or drinks you consume. Even though juices are natural, they contain high amounts of sugar. Whether or not the sugar you consume is natural, your body doesn't know the difference. Sugar is sugar, and your body will react to an excess of it.

**Do**.......... dilute your juices, using about 2/3 juice to 1/3 water. If that's still too strong for you, try 1/2 juice and 1/2 water. Drink small quantities or drink them after you have eaten something, especially if you find that taking them on an empty stomach causes you problems.

**Do**.......... be inventive. Introduce new, unprocessed foods that have no preservatives, additives or chemicals. Look especially for whole grains and vegetables.

47

**Do**.......... arrange food to look palatable.

**Do**.......... broil, bake or steam food.

**Do**.......... attend some natural cooking classes. You will be taught to reduce sugar, salt, saturated fats, cholesterol and allergenic foods from your diet and still enjoy eating. Call your local schools, libraries and health food stores, or scan the local papers to find out what is available in your area.

**Do**.......... understand the meaning of "enriched." It does not mean extra amounts of vitamins. It means a small amount of some of the vitamins that were processed out of the food have been replaced.

**Do**.......... have your family stick to some of the basic principles of your diet. The big NO's for a hypoglycemic (sugar, white flour, alcohol, tobacco and caffeine) are detrimental to anyone's health.

**Do**.......... change your attitude about what constitutes a snack. We tend to think of snacks in terms of goodies or sweet treats. A good snack can be a half-baked potato with broccoli, half-stuffed tomato with tuna fish, some steamed zucchini and onions on a half cup of brown rice, a chicken leg or a slice of turkey.

**Do**.......... seriously consider going to OA (Overeaters Anonymous) or AA (Alcoholics Anonymous). Many HSF members found these meetings to be extremely helpful in controlling their addictions to sugar and food in general.

**Do**.......... be aware of the fact that some medications contain caffeine. If you're having reactions to the following medications, bring this matter to the attention of your physician: Anacin, APC, Caffergot, Coricidin, Excedrin Fiorinal, Four-Way Cold Tablets and Darvon Compound, etc.

**Do**.......... weigh yourself every day. Be aware of weight gain and weight loss. This is vital information in maintaining good health.

**Do**.......... check into other areas if you don't make progress with dietary changes. Hypoglycemia has been linked to allergies, hyperactivity, schizophrenia, juvenile delinquency, learning disabilities and candida albicans. Read the books recommended in the appendix for additional information.

**Do**.......... invest in the *Low Blood Sugar Cookbook*, by Edward & Patricia Krimmell. It can be easily purchased at www.amazon.com

**Do**.......... start a library of cookbooks. They don't necessarily have to be for hypoglycemics. Many good books with no or low sugar recipes are available.

**Do**.......... try at least one new recipe a week. At the end of the year you'll have tasted 52 new dishes, thus, ensuring that you are not tied to eating the same dull fare. It will help you look forward to mealtime and you won't feel so limited with your diet.

**Do**.......... store your food properly to avoid contamination and spoilage resulting from bacteria and molds.

**Do**.......... wash your fruits and vegetables thoroughly to reduce or remove the amount of pesticide residue.

**Do**.......... be aware that chemical sensitivities can aggravate LBS and induce reactions in vulnerable people. Paints, pesticides, solvents, gas stoves, smoke, even perfumes and hairsprays can make some people sick.

**Do**.......... know the seriousness of smoking cigarettes, especially for the hypoglycemic. According to our past Surgeon General, C. Everett Koop, "It is clear that nicotine in cigarettes and other forms of tobacco makes them addicting in the same sense as heroin and cocaine."

**Don't......** panic when you first hear about all the foods that you must eliminate from your diet. Keep repeating all the foods that you CAN eat—there are plenty.

**Don't......** stay on a diet that is not supervised by a professional, whether it's a physician, a nutritionist, or a holistic health practitioner. It should be someone with a degree or some training in nutrition.

**Don't......** forget that being PREPARED with meals and snacks is the key to a successful diet and a healthier you.

**Don't......** be apprehensive about eating out. Many restaurants now have salad bars, making it much easier for the hypoglycemic (just be sure to use either oil and vinegar or lemon juice for dressing). Lean meat, fish, vegetables and salad can be ordered at almost any restaurant.

**Don't......** skip breakfast. It's the most important meal of the day for a hypoglycemic.

**Don't......** worry unnecessarily about weight gain or loss at the beginning of the diet. As long as it is not severe and you are being supervised by a health care professional, it's common to have a weight fluctuation when the body is experiencing dietary changes.

**Don't......** compare your results or progress with anyone else's. Each body's metabolism is different.

**Don't......** take over-the-counter drugs or diet pills unless you have discussed this with your physician. They can have an adverse effect on hypoglycemics.

**Don't......** be obsessive about your diet. The CONSTANT focus on what you can and cannot eat will only instill more fear, stress and frustration.

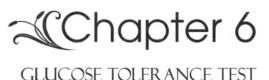

# Chapter 6

## GLUCOSE TOLERANCE TEST

So you think you may have hypoglycemia. You have all the symptoms. After discussing it with your physician, he agrees to give you a glucose tolerance test (GTT) to confirm the diagnosis. A test for three or four hours is requested when diabetes is suspected, but a six-hour glucose tolerance test is by far the most reliable method to detect low blood sugar. You should settle for nothing less.

The night before having the GTT, you will be asked to fast after your evening meal. You are to eat or drink nothing until the time of the test. When you arrive at the doctor's office or laboratory, still fasting, a tube of blood will be drawn and you will be asked to give a urine specimen.

Then, you will be given a very sweet beverage called "Glucola" to drink. This drink contains a measured amount of glucose. Your blood will be drawn in 30 minutes and once again in one hour after drinking the glucola. For each hour after that, you will give a blood sample until five or six hours have passed. A urine specimen is given each time your blood is drawn.

Each tube of blood and each urine specimen is tested to determine the amount of glucose it contains. When the report is sent to your doctor, he or she will be looking for glucose levels above or below normal at any time during the test.

During the test, you may start to sweat, get dizzy, weak or confused. If you experience these symptoms to the point of being extremely uncomfortable, or you get a headache or your heart starts beating quickly, ask the doctor's staff to draw your blood IMMEDIATELY. Any of those symptoms could be a sign that your blood sugar has dropped to a very low level, and you want your doctor to have the lowest readings possible. If you wait until the next hour, your blood sugar may go back up and your doctor will be deprived of information essential to making an accurate diagnosis.

The interpretation of the GTT is just as critical as its administration. Because individuals have different body chemistries, what is a normal drop or curve for one patient may not be for the next. Do not forget that laboratory tests are only aids to a diagnosis, not the final word.

Remember, too, that the test is not for everyone. Children and the elderly, in particular, frequently require another method. Dr. Carlton Fredericks, author of *Carlton Fredericks' New Low Blood Sugar and You*, frequently used "therapeutic diagnosis." "This means putting the suspected hypoglycemic on the correct diet and watching the response. If, after a month or two, the symptoms are significantly reduced, the diagnosis has been established." This procedure can be a less expensive, more convenient and less stressful method for diagnosing low blood sugar.

In conclusion, if you've read the basic facts about the glucose tolerance test, discussed it thoroughly with your physician and both of you have decided that this test is necessary, read the do's and don'ts first.

**Do**.......... understand the purpose, procedure and instructions BEFORE you have the glucose tolerance test administered.

**Do**.......... make sure the test is scheduled first thing in the morning (no later than 9:00 a.m.).

**Do**.......... ask the doctor or nurse to repeat instructions if you do not fully comprehend what you are or are not supposed to do.

**Do**.......... tell your physician, if he/she is not aware, if you are on any kind of medication. Some medications may affect blood sugar levels.

**Do**.......... use the "therapeutic diagnosis" for children and the elderly.

**Do**.......... bring someone with you, especially if you are experiencing severe symptoms.

**Do**.......... bring a book, newspaper or magazine of your choice to help overcome the boredom. Sitting five or six hours is not something we're used to doing. Consequently, restlessness often sets in.

**Do**.......... have a pen and paper available to write down all the symptoms you are experiencing and at what time.

**Do**.......... bring a sweater with you. Very often, a patient will experience chills during the GTT. It is best to be prepared.

**Do**.......... arrange beforehand to have someone pick you up if you go alone for the test. Sometimes, afterward, you may be weak and driving could be difficult.

**Do**.......... bring a snack to eat immediately after the test, particularly if you must go home alone. Eating some protein (nuts, seeds, meat, cheese, etc.) will bring your blood sugar up, allowing you to feel good enough to get home safely.

**Do**.......... set up an appointment before you leave to go over your test results.

◦◦◦◦◦◦◦◦◦◦

**Don't**...... demand a glucose tolerance test. It is not always necessary.

**Don't**...... accept a three or four hour glucose tolerance test for diagnosing hypoglycemia.

**Don't**...... demand to have the glucose tolerance test if you have a fever or infection. It could affect the test results.

**Don't**...... be shortchanged. Go over the results of your GTT with your physician thoroughly.

**Don't**...... be fooled by the terms "borderline" or "mild" in the case of hypoglycemia. Too often when patients hear these terms, they don't take their diagnosis seriously. This could eventually cause grave consequences.

**Don't......** dismiss the fact that you may still be hypo-glycemic even if the GTT doesn't confirm the diagnosis. Laboratory tests are not always con-clusive. The conditions under which the test is given may alter the results. The best rule to follow is: don't treat the results of the test, treat the symptoms.

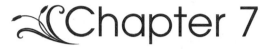

# Chapter 7

## EDUCATION A MUST

L et's pretend it's your husband's birthday and you want to surprise him with his favorite meal; veal cordon bleu. It has been a while since you last made it. You have all the ingredients but just don't remember how to make the stuffing. Now you did have an excellent cookbook—in fact, that's where you got the instructions the first time. You'd better find it.

Your anniversary arrives and you can't believe your eyes. You're overwhelmed by the gift your family bought you—the food processor you always wanted. You just can't wait for a special occasion or holiday so you can show off your culinary skills. However, after you open up the box and see all the pieces, you wonder, "Will I ever learn to use them all? Does this food processor come with a book? It must have directions."

It doesn't matter whether you're whipping up a gourmet meal, fixing a car, planting a vegetable garden or sitting down to learn how to operate a new computer, you need all the information and complete instructions BEFORE you begin.

You need to take the same kind of care with hypoglycemia. Read every book you can get your hands on that discusses the subject. Some will contradict each other, others will be confusing and difficult to understand. No matter, you will learn something from each of them. Remember, too, you don't have to read the thick books all at once, you can read them a chapter, a page or a few paragraphs at a time. Just do it consistently. Learning takes time, energy, patience, and commitment. Don't give up. Just do it gradually and consistently. Don't say you don't have the time or ability, you do.

I wish I could personally introduce you to two HSF members who have taken "don't" out of their vocabulary. First there's Walter. Speak of determination! Here is a man who traveled for more than two and a half hours—EACH WAY —to attend our meetings. Walter was not sure how many miles he traveled because he had to drive very slowly. Otherwise, his 1970 Ford pickup truck might not made it. When I asked him why he made the trip every month, he didn't hesitate to respond, "Because I want to get better. I believe the meetings help me just like Weight Watchers helped my wife. Also, I have a lousy memory, so it's a reminder of what I have to do."

Then there's Hazel. I think she attended almost every meeting the HSF held.

I asked Hazel to share with you why she attended almost every meeting. "I was in terrible condition," she replied, "almost ready to commit suicide. In fact, at one point, I had a knife to my wrist. I threw it down and cried to my husband. . . he had to get me a doctor. I was confused, depressed, shaky. I was so angry because I couldn't do what I wanted to."

"I found a doctor in Beverly Hills. He took a glucose tolerance test but stopped it in the fourth hour because I was passing out. He was the first to tell me I was hypo-glycemic but that I shouldn't worry. He recommended that I just eat candy, hard sour balls every hour, and go to see a psychiatrist. He also handed me the usual one-page diet. I locked myself in the house for a month. I didn't get off the couch. Then one day I read your article in The Miami Herald. Since the diet the doctor gave me wasn't working and I was desperate, I attended the first HSF meeting."

I asked Hazel what the meetings had done for her. "They gave me the courage to stay on the diet," she said. "When I missed a meeting, I found that I would slip off my diet. I also learn something new every time I attended, even if it was only one thing. Sometimes I think I'm well and

61

can do it alone, and then realize that I need support. You not only learn from each other, but you realize you're not alone."

It's not so important what method you use. Books, tapes, lectures — they all give you the opportunity to learn, listen and share. Both Hazel and Walter can attest to this. I hope that one day you will, too.

**Do**.......... educate yourself about hypoglycemia. It is a MUST in order to control your symptoms and make the healing process as painless as possible. I cannot stress enough that KNOWLEDGE AND UNDERSTANDING OF THE CAUSES, EFFECTS AND TREATMENT OF THIS CONDITION ARE IMPERATIVE.

**Do**.......... start by getting a small library of books—at least three—by leading authorities in the field of hypoglycemia. (See the list of recommended books in the appendix). Then make it a habit to re-read them occasionally. You may find it more enlightening and informative on the second or third reading.

**Do**.......... buy yourself a marker and, while reading, mark any sentence that you feel applies to you and that you want to remember for future reference. Perhaps there is a sentence or paragraph that upsets or confuses you, mark it and discuss it with your physician or a health care professional working with hypoglycemic patients. Usually, just a simple explanation clears the way to a healthier you.

**Do**.......... realize that NO book will supply ALL the answers. Some, in fact, will be contradictory. Do take the information you feel you understand and apply it to yourself individually.

**Do**.......... consider tapes. For those who abhor the idea of reading, or who cannot read, for whatever reason, there are tapes available on hypoglycemia. These, fortunately, can be played any where at any time that's convenient.

**Do**.......... you suspect that your child, husband, wife, co-worker or friend is hypoglycemic? Are they reluctant to read any books or listen to tapes? If so, get some brief articles on the subject and leave them around the house, office or in their room. The bathroom mirror or the refrigerator door is an excellent place to start.

**Do**.......... attend meetings, lectures and seminars NOT ONLY on hypoglycemia, but on any health-related subject. Since most illnesses, such as heart disease, cancer, arthritis, diabetes, schizo-phrenia, are now being linked to improper diet, you are likely to get nutritional advice at any meeting you attend.

**Do**.......... your homework. Find out about such meetings through your local newspaper, radio stations, TV (some early morning shows will list meet-ings), cable television, library, physician, health food store, hospital and Chamber of Commerce.

**Do**.......... contact your hospital, library or school. If no health-related meetings are scheduled, particu-larly on hypoglycemia, request that they consid-er the subject. This will alert your area to the needs and wants of the community.

**Do**.......... write down the date and time of the meeting, put it on your calendar, make arrangements with baby sitters, drivers and family members. Explain how important your attendance is at these meetings and prepare to swap services so that feelings of guilt or imposition do not arise.

**Do**.......... take your spouse or an immediate family member with you. It will take some of the pressure off the relationship if they understand the causes of your symptoms.

**Do**.......... use this time to share. If at first you're uncomfortable, try again at another meeting. Sharing experiences often relieves tension and fear, two emotions that can impede progress.

**Do**.......... have questions ready. Most meetings are followed by a question and answer period. Take advantage of this opportunity to gain invaluable information.

**Do**.......... consider attending OA (Overeaters Anonymous) or AA (Alcoholics Anonymous). Even though they may not provide nutritional information per se, they will help you deal with addictive behavior. As hypoglycemics, we are addicted to certain foods—white sugar and white flour are the biggest culprits.

**Do**.......... form your own support group, if nothing else is available. Two, three or four people gathered together, sharing and offering hope, can be the best medicine any doctor could prescribe.

65

**Don't......** pass up any opportunity to help make the journey back to health through information obtained at meetings, lectures and seminars.

**Don't......** give repeated excuses such as: I can't drive at night, it's too far, I can't get a baby sitter, etc. Perhaps the first time these excuses might be valid, but you should prepare for the next time.

**Don't......** surround the speaker before or after the program and try to get a diagnosis. Not only is it unfair to the speaker, but it can do you harm. It is impossible to make a diagnosis without a complete medical history and list of symptoms.

# ʚ℈Chapter 8

## ARE VITAMINS NECESSARY?

In 1984, I decided to leave my business partner, Marge, to give more time to the HSF. Our business was at the peak of its success. She and my husband were appalled that I would bow out, but I knew it was something I had to do.

When we were at the lawyer's office to sign the final papers, she seemed unusually upset. Her speech became slurred, she couldn't concentrate and she appeared lethargic. Her problems got worse and I became more alarmed. Although Marge was only in her mid-30s, she had suffered a stroke two years earlier, and I was worried that it might be happening again.

Questions poured out of me—"Marge, why are you so nervous? Are you angry? Did you take a tranquilizer? Did you have a drink before you came here?" After throwing dozens of questions at her, I discovered the real culprit. Marge suffered from Premenstrual Syndrome (PMS) and was taking vitamin B-6 because she had heard that it could help control her symptoms. She bought a bottle of vitamins and, without knowing the proper dosage, began popping them into her mouth like gumdrops. She was overdosing on her vitamins.

In her effort to relieve pain, Marge, like so many of us, didn't bother to ask questions. She didn't take into consideration the proper dosage, the risk of allergic reactions, and the possible side-effects of combining medications with other vitamins or food. So desperate in her attempt to find a fast and easy cure, she did not even consider the potentially harmful consequences. Marge's poor judgment and inadequate information left her with an apprehensive and fearful decision about ever taking vitamins again.

This story is not unique. Situations similar to Marge's occur much too often. They breed controversy. Therefore, for every published article you read recommending the use of vitamins, be assured you will find a contrary view that discards them as nonessential.

The American Medical Association and the American Dietetic Association claim that if one consumes food from the four basic food groups and obtains the Recommended Daily Allowance (RDA), then the use of vitamins is unnecessary. But, who always eats a balanced diet?

Both associations feel that most Americans can and should get all the nutrients they need to be healthy from food rather than supplements. I don't think any advocate of supplements would disagree. However, what most Americans CAN and SHOULD do are not necessarily what they ARE doing. In fact, due to certain circumstances which I'll soon discuss, most Americans are nutritionally STARVED!! How? Read on.

Many of you have asked the question, "Do I need vitamins?" only to be told to just eat balanced meals. According to television commercials, one would tend to believe that a balanced meal consists of a hamburger, french fries and a coke.

Most of us are on a merry-go-round. Not the one for fun, but a merry-go-round of life; one that leaves us too busy and tired to get off and catch our breath. Many of us are faced with job and financial insecurities, family and marital difficulties, sickness, casualties and even death. It's no wonder that little time is spent on learning about the effects of poor dietary habits. Consequently, the diet of the 21st Century often consists of fast foods, heavily fried, sugar-laden, canned, frozen or leftover meals. Here lies just one of the many reasons why most people do not get sufficient amounts of vitamins and minerals in their diets.

Let's take into consideration some of the other vitamin "robbers:"

air pollution
alcohol
caffeine (coffee and soft drinks)
food additives, preservatives and food coloring
food processing
medication (Diet pills, diuretics, laxatives)
menstruation
soil depletion
stress (mental or physical)
tobacco

Examine the above list and review your dietary habits to see if you are eating a variety of fresh foods. Does your list include fresh vegetables, lean meats, whole grains and fiber?

What cooking methods do you use? Do you broil, steam or bake? How do you store your foods, particularly fruits and vegetables? All of these factors play a role in determining the amount of vitamins and minerals one actually consumes.

So, now, where does all this leave the hypoglycemic? Every book I've read on hypoglycemia and every doctor I've worked with over the past 22 years recommends vitamin and mineral supplementation for hypoglycemics. Vitamin therapy in conjunction with proper diet, exercise and reduction of stress has a positive, supportive and therapeutic effect in the treatment of hypoglycemia.

However, before you swallow that capsule, pill or liquid, read the following do's and don'ts:

**Do**.......... be informed and seek professional advice before starting any long-range, extensive vitamin therapy.

**Do**.......... check out your local osteopathic physician, chiropractor, nutritionist or dietician if your present medical physician cannot supply you with this information. The aforementioned professionals are more likely to incorporate vitamin therapy as an adjunct to the healing process. Make sure the person you consult is licensed. Also try to speak to someone who has already used the practitioner's services and thus can give you insight as to their ethics, reputation and success.

**Do**.......... inform your physician if you are taking vitamins, especially if you are under that doctor's care for a particular disease or condition and/or are taking medication. Some vitamins and medications don't mix well and destroy or weaken each other's effects.

**Do**.......... check out the reputation of the vitamin store where you purchase your vitamins, especially if you're purchasing them without professional guidance. Ask questions about the vitamin or vitamins you are considering, such as: What is the vitamin supposed to do? Should you expect side effects? How long should you take the vitamin? Is there any literature available on the product?

**Do**.......... make absolutely certain that the salesperson's first interest is in your health and safety and not in making a sale. If the salesperson has a forceful approach, leave and look for another store.

**Do**.......... check the price of vitamins. Once you know what you have to take, shop around for the best price.

**Do**.......... double check the dosage you are to take, the time of day it should be taken and any other instructions.

**Do**.......... check vitamin interaction. Avoid taking vitamins with alcohol or medication.

**Do**.......... make sure the vitamins you purchase haven't been tampered with. Check that the label hasn't been broken.

**Do**.......... throw out any bottle whose label you are unable to read, either because it's faded or damaged.

**Do**.......... make sure the vitamins you purchase are not made with any fillers. There should be NO sugar, corn, wheat or starch.

**Do**.......... keep all vitamins in a cool place and keep them out of reach of children.

**Do**.......... take vitamins with meals, unless otherwise directed.

**Do**.......... remember to take your vitamins with you on vacation and business trips. This is usually a time of increasing stress, strong activity and change of diet, and therefore not a good time to discontinue any program you are on.

**Do**.......... STOP taking vitamins if you suspect them to be a cause of nausea, diarrhea, constipation, etc. You can introduce them at a later date, always one at a time. If there is still a reaction, STOP immediately.

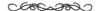

**Don't......** take vitamins indiscriminately! They can be just as harmful as medicine if taken without knowledge and caution.

**Don't......** double up on vitamins, thinking that if one is good, then two must be better. This is not necessarily so. Too many vitamins can be just as harmful as too much medication.

**Don't......** follow anyone else's vitamin program. You should have your own. REMEMBER: everyone is a unique individual with different needs. This individuality includes vitamin therapy of any kind, and therefore should be supervised by a professional.

**Don't......** run out and get the "vitamin of the month." Educate yourself before experimenting.

**Don't......** stop any medication abruptly because you start taking vitamins. Seek professional advice about combining the two.

**Don't......** stock up on vitamins. Your needs may change. Buy vitamins as you need them.

# ᴄ𝒞Chapter 9
## HOW IMPORTANT IS EXERCISE?

Have you ever made a list of things you wanted to accomplish? I don't mean just a to-do list for next Monday, but a laundry list of goals that you want to achieve in your lifetime. I've written at least a dozen of these lists. At one point, I was adding one lifetime goal every day. I soon felt overwhelmed and frustrated because I knew I could not complete them all. I had to stop because I felt oppressed just thinking about the three dozen things I HAD to achieve in my lifetime.

No matter how ambitious my lists became, exercise was hardly ever on them, or if it was, it was near the bottom. This is probably because I was never athletic. I was born in Brooklyn, New York, in a six-family tenement house with no lawn or backyard. The nearest park was miles away. Skating was the only sports activity I participated in. There were plenty of schoolyards, sidewalks and empty streets around, but that was the extent of my exercise as a child.

Some of my friends are still shocked when they hear I don't know how to ride a bicycle.

My attitude about exercise changed many years ago when I attended a health seminar at which Covert Bailey, author of *Fit or Fat?* was one of the program speakers. After hearing him talk on the importance of exercise, I was totally convinced that I had to add exercise to my existing hypoglycemic regimen. I was controlling my hypoglycemia through diet and vitamins, but I knew I could fine-tune my physical condition, improve it, tone and strengthen my body if I incorporated specific daily physical activity into my life.

Now, you mention it and I've tried it—aerobics, yoga, stationary bike, mini-trampoline, jogging, swimming, jumping rope—I've done them all. It was not until May 19, 1986, that I started walking. At first, I walked just a quarter of a mile, then a half mile and then, within a month, I was walking two miles a day, four to six days a week. This was a milestone for me. Walking has since given me more energy and flexibility, relaxes me better than any tranquilizer, suppresses my appetite and rejuvenates me both emotionally and physically.

Hopefully, it won't take you years of procrastination before you incorporate an exercise program into your daily life. Perhaps you can't do it now; you may be experiencing too many hypoglycemic symptoms. However, try making that list of goals as soon as you can. Just don't put exercise at the bottom.

The do's and don'ts of exercise are as follows:

**Do**.......... get your physician's approval before starting any exercise program. Most likely you will be given a complete physical, including an EKG and stress test, depending on your age, medical history and present symptoms.

**Do**.......... seek alternative advice from a health and fitness expert if you choose to ignore the above.

**Do**.......... choose your exercise carefully. The best exercises for hypoglycemics are: walking, swimming, dancing, jumping rope or riding a stationary bike. Walking is the most effective exercise, in addition to being the most compatible with normal daily activities. Depending on the stage of illness you are in, walking is the least stressful exercise for a hypoglycemic. Running, jogging or strenuous aerobic classes should be held off until most of the physical symptoms are controlled.

**Do..........** seek a non-strenuous aerobic exercise program as an alternative to or in conjunction with walking.

**Do..........** make sure the class you choose has an instructor who is qualified through both training and experience.

**Do..........** check for information about time and date of classes, particularly free ones that are advertised in newspapers or community news bulletins.

**Do..........** find a private instructor who will give you personalized lessons if you are afraid to start your exercise program with a group. Use the instructor until you are ready to join a group, which should be in a relatively short period of time. Yes, a personal instructor is expensive, but you will only be using that person for a short time. It is well worth the added expense.

**Do..........** stretch before doing any exercise.

**Do..........** switch exercises occasionally. It avoids over-development of certain muscles.

**Do..........** a slower version of an exercise to warm up or cool down.

**Do**.......... be properly fitted with the appropriate clothing, depending on the exercise and climate. Avoid anything too heavy and tight in summer and too thin and flimsy in winter.

**Do**.......... be properly fitted with shoes.

**Do**.......... check the floor or exercise area for anything hazardous. For example, if you choose to skip rope, make sure the floor is not slippery or wet.

**Do**.......... consider a therapist who does body manipulation or deep muscle massage (osteopath, chiropractor or massage therapist) if sore muscles, malignment of your body or torn ligaments prevent you from exercising. A massage therapist can produce better results than medication, a frequent foe of hypoglycemia.

**Do**.......... consider a "buddy system" if you need support or motivation to start a program. Grab your spouse or friend and begin together to reap the benefits of an alternative method to achieve good health and fitness.

**Do**.......... use every opportunity to increase your activity. Examples: Park in the far corner of the parking lot (during the day only) when shopping or going to work and walk those extra steps; pass up the elevator and take the stairs; and use a stationary bike while watching television.

❧

**Don't......** set high expectations. If you are leading a sedentary life, it would be unrealistic to walk one or two miles at first. You have to build up your stamina SLOWLY.

**Don't......** think you can lose weight quickly by pushing yourself to exercise too frequently. You'll only hinder any program you are on.

**Don't......** push yourself to exercise if you are too fatigued or are experiencing severe symptoms of hypoglycemia.

**Don't......** exercise on a full stomach or exercise on a completely empty stomach, either. Eat an hour before exercising to avoid a blood sugar drop. Remember: don't eat a big meal; you should instead be eating several small meals throughout the day.

**Don't......** walk in hot sun, severe cold, or other undesirable conditions, such as rain, snow or strong winds.

**Don't......** wear tight clothes, especially zippers or buttons if you're in an exercise class where you must lie on your back or stomach.

**Don't......** buy inexpensive shoes In the long run they'll cost you dearly .

**Don't......** compare your progress with someone else's. Each body is unique; therefore, length and success of each program is different.

**Don't......** give up too quickly on any program where you don't see results.  Be PATIENT some programs don't result in a visible improvement for weeks or months.

"I don't want to die. Can I die from
hypoglycemia?"

Dave 1996

# Chapter 10

Y ou found a doctor, took the glucose tolerance test and it's confirmed—you have reactive or functional hypoglycemia. You begin to read about your condition, follow a diet, start on a vitamin program and, to your surprise, have enough energy to begin exercising. Even though your pace and timing may be slow at first, it's something you've never done before.

The severity of your symptoms starts to disappear. You're able to function—go to work, attend school and/or handle home situations. You should be thrilled. But you're not. You're full of fear, guilt and anger, and the loneliness is unbearable. You cry frequently. Discussing your feelings with family and friends only makes matters worse. Too often you hear remarks such as, "You should be grateful you only have hypoglycemia. Luckily, it's not cancer or a disease you could die from."

No, hypoglycemia will not kill you but, according to Dr. Harvey Ross, in his book, *Hypoglycemia, The Disease Your*

83

*Doctor Won't Treat,* it's a disease that will make you wish you were dead.

Is there anything you can do? Yes. Maybe it's time to consider psychotherapy.

Although the attitude about seeking therapy is somewhat better, there are still many myths associated with this approach. At one time, it was considered only for people who were totally out of control, or for the severely mentally and emotionally ill. Consequently, people were afraid to open up, to share their inner most thoughts and secrets. If they did, perhaps some therapist would label them as "crazy," take control of their lives, put them away or do something else equally as bad.

Some people believe that nobody else ever has these feelings so therefore, no one else understands what they are going through. They fear exposing themselves and leaving themselves vulnerable.

Fortunately, for many, this thinking has changed. Today, it's not "Are you going for therapy?" but "Who are you going to?" Therapy, and there are many different types to choose from, has reached a level of acceptance. Some are seeking counseling to prevent minor problems from becoming major ones, some are seeking direction as to where they want to go in life, while others are trying to reclaim their lives entirely.

If you feel mentally and emotionally lost, if the physical problems of hypoglycemia are too much to bear, if you're ready to open up and discover the "real" you, and if you're ready to deal with all of those emotional issues in your life that you have put on the back burner, then therapy may be for you. Therapy does for the mind what diet and exercise do for the body. It's an investment that will pay dividends for the rest of your life.

§

**Do..........** have a physical evaluation and any necessary tests to rule out a physical disease or condition before beginning extensive therapy.

**Do..........** consider seeking therapy when the feeling of "I can't cope" arises. Waiting until an emergency or crisis, may force you into impulsive, short-sighted decisions.

**Do..........** look at therapy as a way to explore and discover yourself, especially if you are depressed and despondent.

**Do**.......... look into the different types of therapy available from psychiatrists, psychotherapists, social workers, hypnotherapists and the clergy. Use the same criteria outlined in Chapter three on choosing a physician.

**Do**.......... be aware that therapists DO NOT have the answers to your problems. One of the things a therapist can do is to help patients trust in their own thoughts and feelings, explore them and follow through in what they really WANT to do and not what they think they SHOULD do.

**Do**.......... search carefully for a competent therapist. Talk to friends. You'll be surprised to find that many are seeking their advice and guidance. Then, without prying into their problems, ask questions: What do they like or dislike about their therapist? Was he or she helpful, and in what way? What beneficial qualities did the therapist possess?

**Do**.......... evaluate the therapist, just as the therapist evaluates you.

**Do**.......... find out:

      1. where the therapist was trained,

      2. the therapist's attitudes and points of view,

      3. how the therapist plans to help you.

**Do**.......... see if you can develop a rapport with the therapist. A trusting relationship between patient and therapist is crucial to the healing process. Ask yourself, "Do I like this person? Am I comfortable? Can I relate freely?"

**Do**.......... realize that the spouse or significant other of the hypoglycemic is under tremendous stress and often needs therapy themselves. According to Dr. Hewitt Bruce, a psychologist in West Palm Beach, Florida, that I have had the privilege of working with both personally and professionally, "No one understands the stress of the spouse or significant other. I believe that more than the patient, the spouse or significant other needs a lot of emotional support. They're not considered sick. They're not considered ill. They're healthy. They are strong. For the spouse it's sometimes a job to care for the hypoglycemic, yet there's no pay, no bonuses, no pat on the back and sometimes no appreciation. So many are suffering emotionally themselves and therapy of any kind could be of great value."

**Do**.......... consider group therapy. Many hospitals have programs to help patients deal more effectively with their emotions.

**Do**.......... remember that in any kind of group therapy confidentiality is crucial. It is the only way TRUST can be established, thus ensuring necessary success.

**Do**.......... check out the new holistic health centers for alternative methods if orthodox treatment fails to help. But be cautious of cultists or quacks.

**Do**.......... check your local papers for support groups that deal with mental or emotional problems.

**Do**.......... be fully aware of all the drastic effects of ECT (Electroconvulsive Shock Therapy), especially memory loss. If you're a computer expert, pharmacist, mathematician, etc., even a slight memory loss can deleteriously affect your life, endangering your livelihood.

**Do**.......... get a second opinion if ECT is prescribed or even suggested. Ask about other forms of treatment and give consideration to there use. Remember—educating yourself about any treatment is crucial.

**Do..........** realize that the end of therapy is, not only as important, but, sometimes more important than its beginning.

**Do..........** read *When To Say Goodbye To Your Therapist*, by Catherine Johnson, Ph.D. It will help you determine whether you are treading water in therapy or whether you can strike out on your own.

⤳⟡⤳

**Don't......** look upon therapy as a sign of weakness. Remember, it takes more strength and courage to admit that you have problems and need help than to ignore the situation.

**Don't......** continue therapy if you feel you're not accomplishing something, even if it's only a small change or a little insight at each session.

**Don't......** blame yourself if:
1. you feel extremely uncomfortable with the therapist,
2. you feel intimidated,
3. the therapist seems judgmental.

**Don't......** go back if the above feelings persist. Don't give up and keep on looking.

**Don't......** stop therapy too suddenly. Give yourself sufficient time for treatment to become effective and gradually, as you grow more confident, wean yourself slowly from the therapist.

**Don't......** become so dependent on your therapist that you won't make a move without his/her direction.

**Don't......** panic if your therapist terminates the relationship. Sometimes, because of a sudden transfer, career change or ill health, your therapist must change his/her venue. Your present therapist should however assure you that they will put you in touch someone just as professional and caring.

# Chapter 11

## POSITIVE ATTITUDE:
## IT WON'T WORK WITHOUT IT

When I first began dreaming about forming the HSF, I was constantly plagued by my own insecurity. I wasn't a doctor, a nurse, or even a college graduate. What made me presume that I could start an organization to help sick people? I didn't have an answer to that question. Yet, there I was trying to form an advocacy group for a disease whose existence medical doctors didn't recognize, whose name most people couldn't pronounce and even fewer could understand.

What was worse, it wasn't even a disease with a lot of drama. It wasn't associated with children or death, and it wasn't even considered life-threatening. As a result, the media covered it only occasionally. How, I kept asking myself, can I make people realize that low blood sugar is real, that the food/mood connection is real, that people can suffer severe emotional problems because their diet has thrown their body's chemistry out of balance?

§

I despaired of ever starting an organization which could have the kind of impact that would make people pay attention, especially because I didn't have any fancy titles or letters, such as Ph.D., after my name. Then, I started to read and re-read. My attitude started to brighten. I found out that many other lay people had contributed to the medical field. People such as Nathan Pritikin, founder of The Pritikin Longevity Center; Jean Nidetch, founder of Weight Watchers; and Barbara Gordon, who wrote *I'm Dancing As Fast As I Can* and told the world about the dangers of Valium in a way no medical textbook ever could.

I knew there was hope. I began to visualize my dreams for the HSF. I wanted support groups in every state, a hypoglycemia hotline, visual aids in schools to warn children about junk foods, and proper testing for people being admitted to state mental hospitals, prisons, juvenile detention centers and jails.

What kept me going, and still does, is enthusiasm, positive thinking, positive people, faith, trust and a firm belief that this is a job that I have to do. It wasn't simple, not at first and not now. But it is getting easier, and it can get easier for you too. The tools, the people, the places, are all there to help. You just have to be ready to receive them. If you can't cope any longer with depression, guilt, fear and denial that a hypoglycemic confronts every day, then do something to replace these negative feelings with positive, uplifting ones.

Start by opening your hearts and minds to Dr. Wayne Dyer's books on positive thinking; Dr. Norman Vincent Peale's on enthusiasm; Norman Cousins' on laughter; and Dr. Leo Buscaglia's on love. Mix them all together and let them be the cement that holds all the other necessary building blocks of good mental health together.

**Do**.......... have a support group of people who won't step on your dreams, who will encourage you, and support you emotionally when you're feeling good AND when you're not.

**Do**.......... have a good selection of positive reading material or tapes. Replacing bad feelings with positive ones is an arduous task. These tapes and books will help do the job when you need an ego boost and no one is around to give it to you.

**Do**.......... put up positive quotes around your house or office. They will lift your spirits and, as a bonus, they'll help lift the spirits of those around you.

**Do**.......... use positive words. Say "I can," "I will," and "I shall." Use only positive phrases, such as "This diet is working. It is the best I've ever had." Repeat these affirmations throughout the day.

**Do**.......... take 15 to 30 minutes every day for meditation or prayer. It refreshes the spirit.

**Do**.......... see happy, uplifting and funny movies. Laughter is terrific medicine.

**Do**.......... try yoga. It lowers blood pressure and relieves stress.

**Do**.......... consider listening to inspirational music, whether it's Bach or the Beatles.

**Do**.......... occasionally treat yourself to something special, whether it is lunch with a friend, a day on the golf course, a manicure, a massage, or a walk in the park.

**Do**.......... put your goals in writing. Read them over each day to instill a sense of purpose and direction. This way, you can check your progress and see that your goals are continuing to be met.

**Do..........** stop procrastinating. If you've put off writing that letter, calling a friend, cleaning out your desk or closet or starting a project, do it NOW.

**Do..........** seriously consider a job change if you've said more than once—"I hate my job." Look into other fields than the one in which you are presently engaged. Learn what the requirements for employment are and take the necessary steps to get the training that's needed for this transition.

**Do..........** seek intellectual stimulation. It enhances the body's immune function and helps increase your vitality. Try reading and/or attending workshops and seminars on varied topics— health, beauty, environment, business, etc. Broaden your horizons and increase your mental acuity.

**Do..........** try to find a teenager, or use your own children, to do extra work around the house or run errands. Remember, you don't have to be Super Mom or Dad! You don't have to do it all—or do it all alone. Share the load of responsibilities. You'll be surprised at how well someone else can do these tasks!

95

**Do**.......... volunteer work. Many times in helping others, we end up helping ourselves.

❧❧❧

**Don't**...... surround yourself with people who have nothing but negative things to say about the world and what you are trying to achieve. They'll only make reaching your goals more difficult.

**Don't**...... use the words "can't" and "won't " Negative words produce negative thinking.

**Don't**...... watch depressing movies or listen to sad music when you feel depressed It will only make you feel worse.

**Don't**...... see problems as obstacles. See them as a way to learn and grow.

**Don't**...... worry so much about the future or dwell on the past that you miss out on "living" today.

# Chapter 12

## HEALTH AND BEAUTY: YOU CAN'T HAVE ONE WITHOUT THE OTHER

I'd like to mention a special someone who, because of her faith and trust in my work and reputation, chose me to assist her for a once-in-lifetime assignment. Carolyn Stein, president of Carolyn Stein & Associates, is a media image consultant. Through her workshops, seminars and keynote speaking engagements, she teaches people how they can create an image of success and develop top communication skills.

Every four years, for the past twenty-four years, Carolyn has been given a very special assignment—media image consultant to the Republican National Convention. For the past three conventions, I went as her assistant.

Carolyn and I met through the Florida's Speaker's Association, of which she and I were both directors. She soon became aware of my previous work in the beauty industry and that I now devoted most of my time and energy to the HSF. It didn't take much persuasion though, for

Carolyn to convince me to go along as her assistant on what was indeed going to be the ultimate "special assignment."

The Republican Conventions I took part in with Carolyn were held in August 1992, in Houston, Texas; August 1996, in San Diego, California; and August 2000, in Philadelphia, Pennsylvania.

Looking back, it's mind boggling to think I had the honor and pleasure of meeting four Presidents and First Ladies, including the Vice President, the Presidents' Cabinet members, Senators, and Representatives from all over the country. Added to that list were stars such as Tanya Tucker, Wynonna Judd, Gerald McRaney, the Gatlin Brothers, Roger Staubach, and Lee Greenwood. At the last convention in Philadelphia, the Rock, Bo Derek, and Rick Schroeder headed the star-studded list.

But it wasn't just our country's leaders or the star-studded list of celebrities that I found so intriguing. It was the participation of today's youth, a large number of very young individuals who weren't home "trying to find them-selves" or just hanging out with friends. They were here in force, with a statement. They wanted to get involved.

Equally impressive were the senior citizens that turned out. Rather than sitting home in front of the television, complain about what is happening in the world, they too took a stand for what they believed and joined in.

So, these two generations along with everyone else, shed their jeans for overalls, for dresses, slacks, shirts, and ties. They put on the outfit to suit the occasion and dove in.

This feeling is beyond politics. It's the very essence of being involved in life and your surroundings. When you commit yourself to life, health and beauty follows. You'll accept nothing less.

I have so many memories and stories of this time. However, one stands out. One evening I was standing in a corridor and I heard a group coming towards me, they were Secret Service Agents, and President Ronald Reagan was with them. Before I knew it, President Reagan was standing in front of me and I was shaking his hand and talking to him! Don't ask me what I said and what he replied. I don't remember, I was so awestruck. But I do remember his presence, his stature, and his demeanor—a giant in history.

Here I was, Roberta Ruggiero. Whether I was meeting leaders of the world, applying make-up, re-doing a hairstyle or straightening out a jacket or tie, I was taking part in American history. It was phenomenal!

However, I kept asking myself, "Why me? Why had I been chosen for this assignment?" Particularly, since most of my work is in the health field. Well, ask a question, and if you stop long enough to listen, there's always an answer.

I have repeatedly said health and beauty go hand and hand. You can't have one without the other. So, there I was, right smack in the middle of proving my theory correct. Everyone with whom I came in contact had a "glow."

I saw skin, hair and nails — all the picture of health. I felt energy, vitality and excitement emanating from everyone. It was evident that the health, beauty, honor, and pride of each individual present would be a contributing factor to the success of these conventions.

The experiences I have had in Houston, San Diego and Philadelphia confirm what I have been saying all along—diet ALONE does not control low blood sugar symptoms. Besides individualizing your diet to meet your particular needs, you must look into a vitamin program, exercise regimen, and stress reduction techniques. You need to maintain a positive attitude, associate with positive people, and look to meditation and prayer for an inner source of peace and fulfillment.

And last, but not at all least, you must look at your physical beauty. It's all there ready to shine. Enhance it a bit with a new hairstyle. Give yourself a facial or a manicure and pedicure. Be daring. Spruce up some old outfits with scarves, pins, fashion earrings or belts. Buy that wild tie you've always wanted or the boots you felt too embarrassed to wear.

Health and beauty walk hand in hand. It's so important to look it, feel it, and be it. Combine the two and you never know where it will take you. It took me to three conventions!

**Do**.......... remember this chapter is to spur you on; to start the wheels going and your enthusiasm flowing. It is just a prerequisite for you to look further into whatever area sparks your interest.

**Do**.......... set a special "beauty" time aside each week just for you. A time to focus and enjoy the art of taking care of your personal needs. A time to pamper yourself from head to toe. You've been worried about what you put INSIDE your body; it's now time to take care of your outward appearance.

**Do**.......... buy some books or magazines on beauty. They will give you more in depth explanations of the areas I've highlighted in the following do's and don'ts. If money is a problem— spend some time at your local library—they usually have the most up-to-date beauty publications.

**Do**.......... start your beauty session with a long, relaxing bath. Light some candles, burn some incense and put on some soft music. Let this be some private time just for you.

**Do**.......... try some aromatherapy in the bath. According to aromatherapist, Gerri Whidden, "Aromatherapy is the use of natural plant essence to produce health, beauty and well being. A few drops of the essences called Essential Oils can be used for inhalation in a bath or as massage oil to stimulate, sedate or uplift."

**Do**.......... try a loofah scrub brush, and use it after soaking in the bath. Wet the loofah with soap and, using a circular motion, massage your skin. It'll remove dry, dead cells and make your skin feel soft as silk. The loofah scrubs are inexpensive and can be purchased at your local beauty supply or drug store.

**Do**.......... give yourself a manicure after a bath or shower. Your cuticles will be soft and easier to push back. First, file your nails GENTLY with an emery board. Take your time to acquire the shape you desire. Make sure that you don't file too much into the nail corners. This weakens the nail.

**Do**.......... push back your cuticles GENTLY and do not use a nail file. Use an orange wood stick. It is even better to cushion the end of the stick with a little cotton. This will allow you to put pressure on the cuticle yet not cause any pain or injury.

**Do**.......... invest in a pumice stone especially designed for the tip of the nail. This will smooth the nail and give you a better looking manicure. Again, this is inexpensive and can be purchased at your local beauty supply store or drug store.

**Do**.......... trim excess cuticles and hangnails CAREFULLY with a cuticle nipper.

**Do**.......... massage your hands with cream. Wipe off the cream that is on the nails. This can be done by using a cotton ended orange wood stick which has been dipped in polish remover. Go over the nail gently, and remove any excess cream or polish.

**Do**.......... apply a base coat. This is absolutely necessary for the nail polish to adhere to the nail. Otherwise, your polish will start to wear off immediately. Then apply two thin coats of your desired color of polish. WAIT as long as you can before applying a top coat. If all these coats of polish are put on without allowing them time to dry between coats, your polish will NEVER fully set.

**Do**.......... apply a soft new shade or try a wild romantic color to your nails, even if you've never done it before. I promise it'll perk you up!

**Do**.......... give yourself a pedicure using the same steps as above.

**Do**.......... treat yourself to a professional manicure and pedicure. Your birthday or anniversary is the perfect time to indulge yourself.

**Do**.......... treat yourself to a professional facial by a licensed aesthetician at least once or twice a year. In between, a minimum of once a month, give yourself a home facial.

**Do**.......... start by choosing the best facial products for you. It's very hard to recommend a product but, again, a licensed aesthetician would be able to help you decide what's best for your skin type and tone. If an aesthetician is not available in your area, go to a cosmetic counter at your nearest department store.

**Do**.......... start with a cleanser that will remove all residue as the first step of your facial.

**Do**.......... follow it with a deep pore cleanser. Remember to be very gentle with your skin. Don't pull or push it.

**Do**.......... use a gentle mask specially chosen for your skin type. Rinse thoroughly. The rinsing process is extremely important. Gently pat dry and use a protective day or night cream.

**Do**.......... remember that consistency is of the utmost importance. Continually starting and stopping any program on health or beauty is most deleterious to your body. It sends mixed signals and can cause undue stress.

**Do**.......... seriously consider a make-up session with a professional cosmetologist. It will enhance your appearance and do wonders for your morale.

**Do**.......... be aware that according to research, cosmetic allergies can also lead to hay fever and asthma. Discuss this with your physician if you feel this may apply to you.

**Do**.......... consider a hair removal process, either waxing or electrolysis, if excess facial or bikini hair a source of discomfort or embarrassment.

**Do**.......... consult a licensed aesthetician in your area for a professional evaluation.

**Do**.......... consider a professional massage. Massage Therapist, Judith McBride, R.N., L.M.T., says, "It is my experience that massage therapy is an excellent way to help nurture and heal others. I have found that by restoring balance through the physical being, the mental, emotional and spiritual self are positively influenced. As a Nurse Massage Therapist, I have effectively blended several disciplines to serve as a natural method for wellness by facilitating healthier lifestyle choices and illness/injury prevention."

**Do**.......... be aware that the benefits of Massage Therapy include: deep relaxation and stress reduction, relief in muscle tension and stiffness, increase in circulation of both blood and lymph fluids and an over-all increase in flexibility and coordination.

**Do**.......... consider a new hairstyle—sometimes a new look is a great image booster and morale ener-gizer. However, remind your hairstylist that you want a hairstyle that is simple, uncomplicated and requires light maintenance.

Do.......... talk to your hairstylist about a permanent. This can add fullness, body and manageability to fly-away, baby-fine or coarse hair.

Do.......... consider cosmetic dentistry—bonding or veneer covering if the appearance of your teeth is causing you shame and embarrassment—or even if you just want to improve your appearance. Seek out professional advice from your local dentist.

Do.......... buy a new item for your wardrobe— a shirt, a blouse, a new tie. Be daring—buy and wear what you've always wanted to wear but were too afraid or ashamed to try. Do it—do it now!

Do.......... put sleep high on your priority list. It's extremely imperative to get a sufficient amount of sleep. It is during the sleep period that the healing process is accelerated.

Do.......... try stress reducing techniques when falling asleep is difficult—deep breathing, meditation, yoga, stretching, or a hot bath. Put on soft music, read a book—whatever kind relaxes your mind, have sex—only if consensual.

**Don't......** sit in the sun and bake because you think a tan will make you look healthy. You'll pay a price— dry, wrinkled skin, plus an increased risk of developing skin cancer.

**Don't......** pull, push, poke or squeeze your skin at any time, especially if you have a blemish on your face. You could cause permanent scarring or accelerate the stretching and aging of the outer layer of your skin.

**Don't......** wear tight clothing, especially belts, shoes or pants. Avoid any unnecessary discomfort.

**Don't......** underdress in winter or cold weather or over-dress on hot summer days. Again we want to avoid severe changes in body temperature.

**Don't......** continue using any make-up or skin care product if you experience any allergic reactions. Consult an aesthetician or dermatologist for advice and direction.

**Don't......** take too hot a bath or soak too long. It could leave you weak. If you're experiencing many hypoglycemia symptoms it is best not to take a bath unless someone else is at home with you in case an emergency arises.

**Don't......** use a sauna, hot tub or jacuzzi unless you use precaution. Please follow posted instructions. If you are experiencing a host of symptoms do NOT use prior to consulting your physician.

**Don't......** have hair removal done—whether waxing, electrolysis or even tweezing—during your menstrual cycle. The outer layer of the skin is very sensitive during this time and often contributes to more pain and sensitivity than usual. If you must tweeze eyebrows—try applying some baby Oragel first—it'll slightly numb the skin and help to lessen the pain. This is an excellent tip for teenagers having their eyebrows done for the first time.

**Don't......** attempt a manicure or pedicure if you have difficult or fungus nails. See a licensed manicurist, pedicurist, or licensed podiatrist.

**Don't......** think for a moment that all of the above do's and don'ts apply only or mostly to women. Today, many men are removing the barrier of "for women only" and enjoying and benefitting from the combination of health and beauty techniques. Be brave men—give some of this a try!

"I can't believe my three-year old was just diagnosed as having hypoglycemia.
I can't stop blaming myself."

Natalie 1999

# Chapter 13

## CHILDREN & HYPOGLYCEMIA
## THEIR UNKNOWN WORLD

Since the HSF's website premiere in 1998, I received an alarming number of e-mails from parents, teenagers and teachers who openly shared their fears, frustrations, and concerns about hypoglycemia. I am including a few of the most notable here so you too can read what these children have been going through. Some of their names have been changed to protect their privacy.

Although their messages are similar, one from Sandra of Cumming, Georgia stands out. Dated October 25, 2000, it opened with this warm acknowledgement of the support we are providing and a request for more information. "Thank you so much for sharing your knowledge and providing a superb web site. There is an area, however, that I found extremely little information and education on and perhaps you can provide enlightenment for those in need. It's in regards to children and hypoglycemia.

"My ten-year-old daughter is intelligent, bouncy and happy most of the time. But over a period of several months, she began to experience significant mood swings, excessive grumpiness, lack of concentration, headaches, etc. Her teacher, my adult friends, and my family related her behavior to "a phase," a lack of sleep, or to the onset of puberty. I finally understood she had hypoglycemia while we were on vacation. One episode in particular was a telltale sign. She was having a major emotional breakdown, which was completely out of character and unsolicited, but within ten minutes of BEGINNING to eat, she turned into a person. Suddenly, the light bulb went off in my head! I am so grateful that I did not simply brush her complaints and symptoms as just life stress or her maturing process."

Sandra had already ordered my book—a good place to start since it is easy to read and understand even for someone as young as her daughter. I stressed the importance of keeping a diet/symptom diary and working with a healthcare professional knowledgeable in treating hypoglycemia and sympathetic to her daughter's needs. I suggested several other books, particularly, *Feed Your Kids Right* by the late Dr. Lenden Smith and *Is This Your Child? Discovering Unrecognized Allergies in Children and Adults* by Dr. Doris Rapp. Both of these authors, leading pediatricians, talk extensively about children, diet and behavior in these books. I also recommended *Food & Behavior: A Natural*

*Connection* by Dr. Barbara Reed Stitt and *Lick The Sugar Habit* by Dr. Nancy Appleton.

Sandra continued to keep me informed about her daughter's progress over the past year and a half, and she has provided insight into what it's like to be a parent struggling to deal with a child who has hypoglycemia. She sent me the following e-mail on March 17, 2002. No book or author on hypoglycemia could have worded it more poignantly, for this comes from the heart and soul of a mother.

"My daughter is doing very well. We are extremely grateful for discovering the root of her problems. There are children struggling physically, mentally and emotionally, and parents are not aware that their food intake is the cause. I grieve to think off all the children being misdiagnosed or medicated that are truly suffering from a blood sugar disorder. I personally believe that because America is addicted to carbohydrates and refined foods, there exists a huge mass of the population that suffers from intermittent or permanent blood sugar disorders. I encourage parents to modify their child's diet as the first line of action to correcting any physical or behavioral problems they see in their children. It may not be the only answer, but will most certainly have a positive affect."

Looking at this problem from an educator's perspective, Janet of Seattle, Washington, wrote, "I am a high school teacher and have a student diagnosed with hypoglycemia. I have a note from her mother asking that high protein snacks be allowed in the classroom to help treat her condition. However, she eats big bags of chips, drinks soda, and yesterday had a big cinnamon roll from the vending machine. She told me, "I need it because I don't feel good." Is this junk food snacking permissible or is it something I should alert her mother to? She has been absent quite a bit this semesters because she has not felt well?"

I commended Janet for her concern and for caring enough to seek a solution. And, of course, my response to her question about junk food snacking was—"No, protein snacks do not consist of bags of chips or a big cinnamon roll. This junk food is exactly what got your student in trouble in the first place."

Fifteen-year old Randy, from Topeka, Kansas, wrote, "I recently found out that I have hypoglycemia. A few days ago I was at school and I just passed out. I was dazed and after I got up, I couldn't see anything for at least fifteen minutes. Should I have more tests? Should I take vitamins? Please send me additional information. I'm just curious about what can happen."

Randy's curiosity is justified. What if he was just a few years older and driving a car when he passed out? What if he felt lightheaded and dizzy while crossing the street or at the top of a flight of stairs? The possible scenarios are endless and most frightening.

I told Randy that I didn't know why the doctor had not insisted on more testing. This was something he and his parents had to ask the physician personally. However, I did explain that reactive hypoglycemia is a result of improper diet, what you are or are not eating. Stress and lifestyle can also exacerbate it. This is the kind of hypoglycemia that the HSF addresses and it sounds like this is exactly Randy's problem. I questioned his eating habits. "Do you have a diet high in sugar? Do you skip meals?" I then recommended that he revisit our website and reread *How To Individualize Your Diet.* I also gave him a list of suggested reading material and told him he could call me if he needed to talk or wanted further direction.

So, where do we go from here? Not every child has hypoglycemia nor should all children be subjected to a glucose tolerance test. However, one in five children in the United States is overweight. That's six million American children! Yes, hereditary, lack of physical activity, and unhealthy eating habits are all contributing factors. But consider this: Americans consume over one hundred and eighty pounds of sugar per person per year! SUGAR and a high sugar diet are the biggest culprits in hypoglycemia. Soda, fruit juices, candy, ice cream and high sugar coated cereals are the norm for today's children. With preteens and teenagers, parents must also consider alcohol and tobacco experimentation. These two substances, when combined, can be very volatile.

If your child is experiencing any of the symptoms that Sandra's daughter, Janet's student, or Randy described, they too may be suffering from hypoglycemia.

A quick recap...mood swings, severe fatigue, insomnia, sudden outburst of temper, failing grades, sleeping in class, and fainting spells are all possible warning symptoms or signs.

The message is loud and clear. Parents, teachers, and community leaders must all band together to help our children. To understand and learn more about the food/mood connection, start with the following simple do's and don'ts.

**Do**.......... open up lines of communication with your child concerning their food habits and possible associated signs & symptoms. Let them know also that wrong choices, even in diet, may produce negative consequences.

**Do**.......... EDUCATE yourselves! Parents, it is your responsibility to be educated in this correlation between diet and behavior. What your child eats and doesn't eat directly relates to how he thinks, feels, and acts.

**Do**.......... search the Internet, local library, bookstores and attend any seminar on this or related subjects. The more you know the better you will be to make an informed decision.

**Do**.......... work with a health care professional that is knowledgeable with hypoglycemia and sympathetic to your child's needs. Re-read the chapter, "How To Find a Physician."

**Do**.......... work with local schools, teachers, counselors and community leaders. Share the information in this chapter with all of them.

**Do**.......... cultivate an on-going relationship with your child's teacher concerning diet and behavior. Open, honest communication is crucial.

**Do**.......... review your child's dietary habits before administration of any medication, especially, Ritalin. Share your finding with his/her physician. Often a change in a high sugar diet will eliminate the need for such hyperactivity medications or minimize the dosage required.A few weeks or months of trying a diet change first could save years of unnecessary medication.

**Do**.......... monitor the amount of junk foods you child is eating. A parent said that his child hid candy wrappers all over the bedroom—under the beds, in his dresser draws, and pants pockets. This is a sure sign of a junk food/candy addict.

**Do**.......... evaluate your child's eating habits, keep a diet/symptom diary and eliminate the big offenders: sugar, caffeine, tobacco and alcohol. A good place to start is by reading the chapter "How To Individualize Your Diet."

**Do**.......... make shopping for food, planning meals, and cooking a family affair.

**Do**.......... read labels carefully. Eliminate any foods or drinks with a high sugar and caffeine content.

**Do**.......... opt for organically grown and pesticide-free products, especially if your child is known to have food allergies. You can even help children start their own vegetable garden. If you live in a city or an apartment, encourage an herb garden, which is smaller and much easier to keep.

**Do**.......... encourage your child/adolescent, or teenager to share any physical symptoms with you. Naturally, if you have a family physician, he/she should also be the first person that should be made aware of severe fatigue, insomnia, panic attacks, fainting spells, etc.

**Do**.......... realize the importance of carrying your Health Emergency Card with you (or your Child) at all times. This card is available from HSF; the order form is at the back of the book. This is especially crucial if anyone has a history of fainting spells. This card includes the emergency telephone number of parent or close relative/friend and physician. Most importantly, it explains that one is hypoglycemic, so paramedics or other health professionals can quickly administer the appropriate medical treatment.

**Do**.......... encourage your child to share any emotional symptoms with parent, physician, close adult, teacher or school counselor, especially depression and suicidal thoughts. If this is not possible, let him/her know that there are anonymous hot-lines available. Check your local yellow pages.

**Do**.......... eat breakfast. It is the most important meal of the day.

**Do**.......... be aware of the harmful dangers in water fasts or diet pills, especially if the latter is taken without a doctor's supervision.

**Do**.......... exercise. Take advantages of opportunities at work or school to join a sports team, take part in gymnastics. If this is not possible, walk or do yoga to relax, anything that gives you some exercise each day.

**Do**.......... forget the soda, go for bottled water. Each 12-ounce bottle of soda has 10 teaspoons full of SUGAR!!

**Do**.......... choose broiled or baked chicken and salads if you must opt for fast foods.

**Do**.......... experiment with high protein bars and shakes, especially if you skip meals. Be aware however, that many bars contain a high amount of sugar. You must read labels.

**Don't......** ignore lack of self control, angry outbursts, hysteria, inability to handle changing or stressful situations. This applies to both adults and children.

**Don't......** assume that children's junk food habits are something they will outgrow.

**Don't......** assume that children understand the importance of good dietary habits. They learn from what they see and hear from other family members.

**Don't......** forget to include a daily multi-vitamin/mineral as part of your child's daily regimen.

**Don't......** put your child on any medication for behavior, particularly for Attention Deficit Disorder (ADD) or Attention Deficit Hyperactivity Disorder (ADHD) without talking to a healthcare provider, evaluating their eating habits, checking for food allergies and food sensitivities.

**Don't......** STOP ANY MEDICATION WITHOUT THE ADVISE OF YOUR PHYSICIAN.

**Don't......** tolerate any doctor who ignores your concerns or your child's symptoms.

**Don't......** forget to be supportive and HUG your children. Let them know that their problems are important to you and that you will always be there to help.

*Especially for teachers:*

**Do..........** have information about diet and behavior available for your students and parents including specific organizations, support groups, and toll free numbers.

**Do..........** in-house educational programs that include students, parents, and teachers.

**Do..........** evaluate the food, snacks and soda that is available to the children, whether in the school cafeteria or vending machines. Challenge their presence and lobby to have any offending food or drink product changed!! Involve other parents and teachers.

**Do..........** be sympathetic if a child and his/her parent inform you that they have a blood sugar management problem and need to have a snack at certain times of the day. Please don't dismiss this request. A snack can be something as simple as a few almonds or a protein bar. This shouldn't disturb the class or other children. You could even use this as an excuse to explain proper diet and nutrition to children. No one, hypoglycemic or not, needs sugar and refined foods and junk food.

**Do**.......... get a written note from a health care professional if you suspect a child may be having a sugar management problem. Or request a parent conference and share what you know. They may be at their wits' end and this information could help them immensely.

"My doctor told me to just eat the candy bar
to raise my blood sugar.
I'd rather have gumdrops."

Suzanne 1998

# 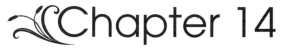Chapter 14

## HYPOGLYCEMIA & ALCOHOLISM
## IS THERE A CORRELATION?

A lcoholism. No one is immune to it. It doesn't discriminate on the basis of race, religion, gender, or socioeconomic status. Sadly enough, there are also no age barriers. Whether it is used as a chemical, drug or food, 23 million Americans are under its influence.

§

From the womb to the grave, alcohol's effect on the body can be devastating. Its physical and emotional effects can range from upsetting the metabolism and nutritional state of the body to increasing the risk of cancer, liver and heart disease, high blood pressure, and diabetes. It can cripple the emotions with low self-esteem, and promote feelings of isolation, rejection, loneliness, hopelessness, and fear.

There is an abundance of literature that indicates that alcohol consumption during pregnancy can put the unborn child at risk for numerous health problems. Even if the child appears unscathed by a pregnancy where alcohol was used, this "healthy" child still has a 30 percent chance of trying alcohol by the time they are nine years old!

Children, who make it through high school without experimenting with alcohol, may not resist the temptation though college. And along with the risk of alcoholism, consider these alarming statistics from the National Institute on Alcohol Abuse and Alcoholism, a division of the National Institutes of Health (NIH). "An estimated 1400 college students are killed every year in alcohol-related accidents, drinking by college students contributes to 500,000 injuries, and 70,000 cases of sexual assault or date rape. Also 400,000 students between 18 and 24 years old reported having unprotected sex as a result of drinking."

Information on alcoholism and treatment options is available just about everywhere—in newspapers, magazines, on the Internet. The problem is so pervasive and devastating that individuals, communities, and businesses have come together to try to combat and educate people about the disease. Three organizations—Business Against Drunk Drivers (BADD), Mothers Against Drunk Drivers (MADD), and Students Against Drunk Drivers (SADD)—are involved with educating the public about the deadly combination of drinking and driving and advocating for harsher laws for offenders. And of course, the most well known organization helping people cope with alcoholism is Alcoholics

Anonymous, which has been providing education and assistance for years.

It would seem that all the information we want about alcohol use/abuse is right at our fingertips. Unfortunately, most of this information fails to acknowledge the connection between hypoglycemia (low blood sugar) and alcoholism. Fortunately, I have managed to compile a small library of texts establishing a correlation between these conditions.

In *Dr. Atkins' New Diet Revolution,* Dr. Atkins writes, "Experience shows that, when an alcoholic succeeds in getting off alcohol, he usually substitutes sweets. This is because almost all alcoholics are hypoglycemic, and sugar provides the same temporary lift that alcohol once did."

Dr. Harvey M. Ross, in *Hypoglycemia: The Disease Your Doctor Won't Treat,* Dr. Ross states "What is most important is the plethora of doctors and counselors who ignore the results of the research that prove that the alcoholic has a blood sugar problem."

According to Dr. David Williams, author of *Hypoglycemia: The Deadly Roller Coaster,* "To combat alcohol and other drug abuse, abstinence, proper diet, nutritional supplementation, and education about abuse and hypoglycemia must be part of the program."

127

Dr. Joan Mathews Larson, author of *Seven Weeks To Sobriety:The Proven Program to Fight Alcoholism Through Nutrition,* has a phenomenal website: www.healthrecovery.com. Acquainting yourself with this incredible resource is a must! Both in her book and website, you will be introduced to Dr. Larson's Health Recovery Center and her in-depth explanation of hypoglycemia and its relationship to alcoholism.

The biggest contributor though to my education on the hypoglycemia-alcoholism connection has been Dr. Douglas M. Baird, Medical Director of the HSF. In our meetings and seminars, Dr. Baird has often reiterated, "I have never, ever seen an alcoholic who was not hypoglycemic. It just doesn't occur, it's the same problem."

Dr. Baird's interest in the treatment of alcoholism dates back to the late 1970's, when he became intrigued by the withdrawal symptoms that many times accompany the cessation of drinking—tremor, weakness, sweating, increased reflexes, gastric symptoms and seizures. In extreme cases people withdrawing from alcohol might even experience visual or auditory hallucinations. These symptoms, he said, often prevented alcoholics from quitting or caused them to replace alcohol with sugar, high carbohydrates, caffeine and/or tobacco (nicotine).

Working on the premise that alcoholism, like hypoglycemia,

was related to a faulty metabolism, Dr. Baird set out to design a program to meet the recovering alcoholic's needs. Preliminary physical and dietary evaluations are completed as well as blood and sugar testing. The chemical imbalance created by years of poor dietary habits is then brought back into alignment with implementation of an individualized diet and vitamin therapy. Dr Baird has been using his program for over 20 years and has a 75 percent success rate in helping alcoholics cope with their disease and not fall into hypoglycemia. His program works, he says, because, "it stabilizes the alcoholics blood sugar and thus makes it easier for the alcoholic to maintain abstinence."

The following e-mail was sent to Dr. Baird from a recovering alcoholic:

"I was diagnosed with severe hypoglycemia in the late 1960's. I am afraid to say that I never really took this condition very seriously until now and only followed the recommended diet for about a year. I have to confess that while I was on the high protein/low carbohydrate diet, with the elimination of sugar & caffeine, I never felt better in my entire life. A new relationship and lifestyle change is what triggered my old eating habits.

"I happened to notice in your bio that you seem to suspect a direct correlation between alcoholism and hypoglycemia.

I also am a recovering alcoholic. While I was in rehab, this was a question that I presented to the doctor attending me. He did not give me any concrete answers.

"I suppose the logical portion of my brain would con-clude that, of course alcoholism is related to hypoglycemia. How could one drink all that sugar and not have "reactive" hypoglycemia? I do know that while in the grip of a heavy drinking binge, I could almost sense that I'd reach for more alcohol in a desperate effort to stabilize my sugar level and it became a viscous cycle. Try to drink more to keep the sugar level from falling too dangerously low and steady myself from shaking so violently.

"I am struggling right now, desperately trying to get myself back on the right path, but seeming to lack the necessary self-discipline. I have even had talks with myself trying to convince myself that this is very, very serious and in order for me to feel better, I have got to muster the determination to give up all the junk that is making me so ill. I have struggled (especially the past three years) with depression/anxiety/insomnia and I am tired of dragging myself through every day feeling exhausted."

It took great courage to write and share the above experiences. It's clear that in this case, hypoglycemia was not taken seriously. Doctors often don't have the answers to the questions we ask and many times we have to find the answers within ourselves. Even with self-discipline and determination, this writer struggled every day. I wonder if she/he had the information contained in this chapter, plus the following do's and don'ts, would the road to recovery had been easier and less painful. I truly believe so.

**Do**.......... EDUCATE yourself thoroughly on the correlation between hypoglycemia and alcoholism by reading *Seven Weeks To Sobriety: The Proven Program to Fight Alcoholism* by Dr. Joan Mathews Larson and *Under The Influence* by Dr. James Mylam.

**Do**.......... look into the work by Dr. Barbara Reed Stitt, author of *Food and Behavior*. Stitt, a former Chief Probation Officer, writes about her years of research and experience with correcting behavior by modifying diet.

**Do**.......... set an example if you are a parent. We cannot tell our children to "just say no to drugs," if we ourselves are not role models.

**Do**.......... make sure your children are supervised, the greatest risk occurs when children are left alone.

**Do**.......... get your child involved with after school activities.

**Do**.......... recognize the warning signs of alcohol and drug abuse in children: decline in grades and school attendance; discipline problems; changes in attitude, friends, and physical appearance; and most importantly, physical conditions such as loss of appetite, excessive fatigue, and sleeping habits.

**Do**.......... recognize the warning signs of alcohol abuse in adults: personality changes, high absenteeism on the job, low productivity, confrontations at work and home, and increase sleeping habits.

**Do**.......... recognize that most, if not all, alcoholics are hypoglycemic and unless both are addressed, recovery is severely hampered.

**Do**.......... realize that recovering alcoholics often replace addiction with some form of sugar, caffeine and/or tobacco (nicotine).

**Do**.......... find a physician, mental health provider, support group (facility if needed), or buddy system that encourages proper nutrition and supplementation with vitamins and minerals.

**Do**.......... insist on appropriate testing (glucose tolerance test, vitamin/mineral analysis, etc.) to determine if you have hypoglycemia.

**Do**.......... reread chapters on "How To Individualize Your Diet," keep a diet/symptom diary, evaluate dietary habits, and eliminate offending foods.

**Do**.......... reach out and ask for professional help. Medical and psychological assistance may be needed more than tough love.

〜〜〜〜〜

**Don't**...... think you can solve your problem ALONE if you are both hypoglycemic and alcoholic. Medical and nutritional therapy and/or guidance are needed.

**Don't**...... be fooled by the temporary high that alcohol gives you. A drop in blood sugar will soon follow this quick-energy feeling resulting in the high/low scenario very familiar with hypoglycemia and alcoholism.

**Don't**...... be ashamed about your addiction. Both hypoglycemia and alcoholism are medical disorders compounded by chemical imbalances and nutritional deficiencies.

133

"There are 39 people in my family with sugar
problems. Some have diabetes,
some hypoglycemia.
It will be a blessing to get help."

Ramona 2002

# Chapter 15

## HYPOGLYCEMIA: A PRELUDE TO DIABETES

It is rare that I have a conversation about hypoglycemia that the subject of diabetes doesn't come up. The thousands of letters and e-mails I've received over the past twenty-plus years confirm that this is a major concern.

One such e-mail, sent in mid-1998 gives you an indication of what I mean. A full time college student at Tulane University in New Orleans writes, "I feel like I'm going to die from this thing that grossly interferes with my life...I want to know everything...I don't understand much. Should I just eat everything when I have an attack? Tell me what to eat when I'm freaking...I also want to know how this affects my metabolism? How does it differ from diabetes? Is it the predecessor? What are the long-term effects? Can this kill me? Because sometimes I want to die or just be able to stick an insulin needle in my arm and feel better. Perhaps it is because I am uneducated on the issues, but it seems to me that diabetics have it easier. They can just "get a fix" so to speak. I don't really like needles but I could get used to them if it would make me feel better, feel normal."

On March 16, 1999 the following came from DM, "I was just diagnosed with hypoglycemia. Can you explain in plain language that I can understand how hypoglycemia is pre-diabetic? Please tell me this isn't true and if so how could I become diabetic?"

It was difficult to respond to these two e-mails. What do you say to someone who sounds so desperate and helpless? Is information enough? In both these cases however, information is THE only answer. When fear and panic sets in because of the unknown, every physical symptom becomes magnified. If only they read *Lick The Sugar Habit* by Dr. Nancy Appleton, *Hypoglycemia: The Classic Healthcare HandBook* by Jeraldine Saunders, or *New Low Blood Sugar and You* by *Dr. Carlton Fredericks*. Each of these books would have answered all the above questions! It saddens me that this information isn't readily available through the medical community. Maybe it is because hypoglycemia and diabetes are neatly separated as health conditions—one is accepted while one is virtually ignored. Hypoglycemia is often only spoken of in the context of insulin and blood sugar level management for people with diabetes.

Just scan your local newspaper and magazines, diabetes (high blood sugar) definitely takes center stage in medical headlines. Right now, Type two diabetes, like obesity, is at epidemic proportions in the United States and the world. Seventeen million Americans have diabetes with 800,000 new cases each year. Is there any wonder why this disease is the fourth leading cause of death? Diabetes also increases the risk of heart disease, gangrene and limb amputation, kidney failure, and blindness. As a leading killer, it also decreases your life expectancy. The saddest part is that 50 percent of those affected may not be aware that they have this deadly disease.

Hypoglycemia (low blood sugar) on the other hand has taken a back seat. There may be an article here, a book there, but seldom do you see statistics. Too bad, for maybe if we had numbers, more Americans would stand up and take notice of its alarming rise. One book I read estimates that 100 million Americans are hypoglycemic. Unfortunately, there are few formalized studies on hypoglycemia as a stand-alone condition. Therefore, it is very difficult to substantiate these numbers. Often, the only research to be found on hypoglycemia is within the context of other diabetes studies.

Because of this however, we may never know how many Americans are suffering, needlessly, from hypoglycemia. Do we need numbers to show that there is a connection between low blood sugar (hypoglycemia) and high blood sugar (diabetes)? Or do we just need to read more of the e-mails that the HSF receives?

"I was diagnosed with borderline hypoglycemia in 1999. My doctor told me not to worry and handed me a single sheet of paper with some diet instructions. Since he didn't seem concerned, I left with the feeling like my condition was "no big deal." I kept eating all my chocolate chip cookies and gave in to all my cravings. I am now dealing with the consequences. I feel terrible. My symptoms are worse and I was just diagnosed (2002) with diabetes. Both my mother and grandmother had diabetes. Why didn't I take this more seriously? What can I do now?"

"I desperately need to find a doctor that knows how to treat my hypoglycemia. My present one told me all I had to do was carry a candy bar with me. My Dad is severely diabetic and I don't want to end up with that disease. I live in the Cincinnati, Ohio area, please help me."

"Can uncontrolled hypoglycemia result in diabetes?"

I asked Dr. Lorna Walker, the HSF's nutritionist, to answer the last question. This was her response. "Hypoglycemia is a blood management disorder in which the pancreas reacts to a rapid rise in blood glucose levels by secreting too much insulin. While in diabetes, when blood sugar gets abnormally high, the damaged pancreas is unable to bring it down by secreting too little. In some cases, this hyper-insulinism is the precursor to adult onset diabetes (type 2 diabetes). The hypothesis is that the overactive pancreas, when predisposed by genetics, diet, and lifestyle finally begins to wear down and the end result is diabetes."

No letter, e-mail or explanation can be as profound as the simple black and white facts. So, in 1998, I added a hypoglycemia/diabetes questionnaire to our website. Due to the increase of questions and concerns about a possible connection between hypoglycemia and diabetes, I wanted to find out if this association could be observed. The goal was to determine whether untreated hypoglycemia is a precursor to diabetes. The survey was also designed to gather information on how and by whom hypoglycemia had been diagnosed and what type of treatments, if any, were found to be beneficial. As this book goes to press, the HSF has received over 5500 responses (3,752 confirmed hypoglycemics) from 25 countries!

We are in the process of sorting through this extensive volume of information to categorize and evaluate the results. Below, however, is a brief synopsis of what we've discovered so far.

**Sixty-four** percent of confirmed hypoglycemics (diagnosed by a physician with a glucose tolerance test) indicated that one or more family members had been diagnosed with diabetes!

With this information, we can alert hypoglycemics to the seriousness of this condition, as diabetes will almost certainly be the next stage if left untreated. It is also critical for diabetics to share this information with other family members as a preventative measure.

When we asked those surveyed what kind of symptoms they experienced, the most common were:

| | |
|---|---|
| Heart Palpitations | 80% |
| Dizziness | 79% |
| Mood swings | 77% |
| Headaches | 74% |
| Depression | 67% |
| Addiction to sweets | 62% |
| Extreme fatigue | 52% |

When diagnosed with hypoglycemia, only 59% changed their diet. That number is high considering only 48% of physicians who diagnosed hypoglycemia, through a glucose tolerance test, recommended treatment. A little more than 50% of the participants incorporated vitamins and exercise while only 25% changed their mental attitude towards the illness. Unfortunately, 23% considered candy the cure-all for their low blood sugar problems.

Check out our hypoglycemia/diabetes survey on our website, www.hypoglycemia.org. It will give you an idea of what we are looking for and how this information will help future treatment of these conditions. This survey of course isn't the answer, as it cannot take the place of medicine or well-structured clinical trials. However, it is actually giving us the questions we need to encourage more scientific research into this condition that is so often not taken seriously.

Before the future, let's look one more time at the present. Diagnosing and managing hypoglycemia is one of the key determining factors in the subsequent development of adult onset (Type 2) diabetes in later life. Diet, lifestyle, age, pre-disposition, and insulin and tissue resistance are all variables that need to be addressed concerning this issue. To date, there is nothing we are able to do to counteract the effects of either aging or genetic pre-disposition. The remaining elements, however, can be managed. If one is successful, there is a good chance that Type 2 diabetes can be prevented or delayed.

Look carefully at the following do's and don'ts. Hopefully, they will encourage you to take action. Making smart dietary choices can make all the difference between staying healthy or becoming chronically ill. In this case, it may prevent hypoglycemia from turning into diabetes. Know that hypoglycemia is real, "it is not a fad disease" as some physicians states it is. It is a blood sugar management disorder and not just a complication of diabetes.

**Do**.......... evaluate your dietary habits if you experience any of the following symptoms:severe fatigue, depression, insomnia, heart palpitations, crying spells, craving for sweets, cold hands and feet, etc. See the chapter "Definition of Hypoglycemia" for complete list of symptoms.

**Do**.......... eliminate the big offenders: sugar, white flour, alcohol and tobacco. See chapter on "How To Individualize Your Diet".

**Do**.......... find a health care professional that is knowledgeable with hypoglycemia and sympathetic to your needs.

**Do**.......... know the definition and warning signs of Type 2 diabetes, the kind that we are addressing here in this chapter. This type of diabetes is usually a result of diet and lifestyle. Common symptoms are unusual thirst, frequent urination, blurred vision and fatigue.

**Do**.......... learn more about diabetes; its causes and effects. Visit the American Diabetes Association's website at www.diabetes.org.

**Do**.......... follow the basic diet guidelines for hypoglycemia if you have been diagnosed as diabetic: NO sugar, white flour, alcohol, tobacco and caffeine.

**Do**.......... work with a nutritionist or diabetic counselor. However, be leery if anyone says that sugar and white flour are OK to eat.

**Do**.......... monitor your blood glucose closely. This is absolutely necessary for diabetics. Some hypo-glycemics also feel that this is helpful and necessary. The medical community hasn't advocated it for the latter.

**Do**.......... increase physical activity.

**Do**.......... control your weight. This is most important since excess weight makes the body less sensitive to insulin, the hormone needed to control glu-cose levels in the blood.

**Do**.......... take diabetic medication if diet, weight control and exercise don't lower your blood sugar levels to normal range. Of course, this is strictly under the care of a physician

**Do**.......... keep blood pressure and cholesterol under control since people with diabetes are more prone to heart disease and stroke.

⸎⸎⸎⸎⸎⸎

**Don't......** make any changes in diet and medication if you are diabetic. Changes must be made under the supervision of you physician.

**Don't......** delay notifying your physician if you feel your diabetic medication has unpleasant side effects.

**Don't......** STOP any medication without the your physician's approval.

# ⁊⟨Chapter 16

## ASK THE EXPERTS

While moving in the summer of 2001, I found myself with 48 boxes labeled "HSF." Since the fall of 1977, I collected over 400 files including hundreds of books and tapes relating to hypoglycemia and The Hypoglycemia Support Foundation, Inc. The cry for help was overwhelming. The boxes contained handwritten cards and letters, lengthy e-mails, notes about desperate telephone calls I had received. Parents, teenagers, boyfriends, wives, husbands; they all had questions they hoped and prayed the HSF could answer.

And answer we did! Dr. Douglas M. Baird, the HSF's Medical Director, and our Nutritionist, Dr. Lorna Walker, addressed the medical questions. Their dedication was extraordinary, their unselfish donation of their time and expertise went above and beyond anything I expected. I responded by sharing my own experiences and what I had learned over the past years.

The information contained in these archives is so valuable that I am including it here. I asked other members of our Medical Board to share their thoughts on the questions posed to us: Dr. Herbert Pardell, Dr. Nancy Appleton, Dr. Stephen J. Schoenthaler, and Nutritional Biochemist Jay Foster. Dr. Nancy Steinman, a psychologist at Miami Heart Institute, also shared her expertise. Without their dedication, caring and concern, this chapter would not have been possible. We extend a very special thank you to all of them.

*(The opinions expressed by the experts should not be construed as a specific diagnosis or treatment recommendations. These answers are offered to provide a framework of information concerning commonly asked questions. Likewise, the HSF does not endorse specific products, tests, or protocols. The HSF encourages each person to take the individual steps necessary to establish the correct diagnosis and treatment regimen.)*

Q. What is the difference between functional and reactive hypoglycemia?

A. Functional hypoglycemia refers to decreases in blood sugar that cannot be explained by any known pathology or disease. It's a nice way of saying, "Your glucose regulating mechanisms aren't functioning normally, and we don't know why." Reactive hypoglycemia refers to hypoglycemia resulting from the body's abnormal response to rapid rises in blood glucose levels caused by diet or stress. The terms are now frequently interchangeable. *Dr. Douglas M. Baird.*

Q. What should I eat when my low blood sugar hits? Orange juice? A candy bar?

A. The worst thing you can eat when your hypoglycemia "hits" is sugar in any form! It may make you feel better temporarily, but soon afterwards your pancreas will over secrete insulin, which caused your blood sugar to drop in the first place. Eating small, frequent meals that are low in fat and carbohydrates and contain moderate amounts of protein is the best way to control your blood sugar. Over time, you will learn what works best for you to keep your sugar within a reasonable range. *Dr. Douglas M. Baird.*

Q. Will hypoglycemia go away?

A. Not really. Blood sugar management disorders are hereditary, and as of this writing, we are not advanced enough to change our genetic code. However, hypoglycemia can be managed and controlled. What this means is that with dietary therapy and lifestyle changes, the number and severity of low blood glucose occurrences can be reduced or even eliminated over time. If a hypoglycemic returns to his/her old eating habits and lifestyle, symptoms will quickly return. Also, when we find ourselves under increasing stress, we are more apt to develop symptoms in those areas where we are weakest, with blood sugar abnormalities being no exception. *Dr. Douglas M. Baird.*

Q. Diabetes runs in my family. Will I have the same sort of problems?

A. Not necessarily. From a genetic standpoint, your predetermined diseases are largely a function of the luck of the draw. Whose genes you inherit determine your susceptibility to many diseases. It must be remembered that genetic predisposition does not necessarily guarantee that you will develop the disease. Blood sugar management abnormalities, which often manifest themselves as hypoglycemia, need not degenerate into full-blown diabetes. These disorders can be managed so that one can minimize the effects of one's genetic inheritance. *Dr. Douglas M. Baird.*

Q. I get heart palpitations, and extensive testing confirms that nothing is wrong with my heart. My diet is not perfect, but could this be the problem? Could hypoglycemia be the culprit?

A. Heart palpitations can be caused by a number of conditions, and many times, we cannot pinpoint the cause. If primary cardiac conditions have been ruled out (and I assume that the usual suspects-stimulants, allergens, etc., particularly caffeine-have been eliminated) but the symptoms are bothersome enough to warrant additional investigation, hypoglycemic episodes could be triggering palpitations and/or tachycardia (rapid heart rate).

Since dietary management is the cornerstone for the management of hypoglycemia, I would suggest that one way for you to determine if there is a connection is to change the way you eat. Remove all refined sugars from your diet, and eat small, frequent meals high in low-fat protein and moderate in complex carbohydrates. Try eating a small protein snack before retiring, but do not overeat.

Remember, dietary manipulation, vitamins, minerals and lifestyle changes are almost always part of an overall treatment program necessary to achieve control of any hypoglycemic symptoms, heart palpitations included. *Dr. Douglas M. Baird.*

Q. My husband quit drinking and now craves chocolate.

A. This is not an uncommon response. Alcohol is simply a very refined sugar. When one quits one form of sugar, they many times substitute another. I have never seen an alcoholic that was not hypoglycemic. Alcohol and sugar are different forms of the same fuel. The inability to properly manage blood sugar levels in the bloodstream may cause a variety of problems, especially with brain function. This can be quite serious. The problem of proper and adequate fueling of the brain must be managed on an ongoing basis if an individual is to function optimally. *Dr. Douglas M. Baird.*

Q. Can having severe hypoglycemia give a false (high) blood alcohol level with a Breathalyzer?

A. When one's blood sugar gets too low, the human body has a number of compensatory mechanisms that will try to correct this condition. One of those processes is called gluconeogenesis, literally "making new sugar." One of the byproducts of that process is acetone. This is the reason why people with blood sugar problems and those on calorie restrictive diets have what the medical profession calls "acetone breath." Law enforcement personnel often confuse this smell with alcohol.

Now, whether the Breathalyzer can discriminate between acetone, other ketones, and alcohol is the critical question. Your attorney will have to contact the manufacturers of that technology to see whether that discrimination can be made by the available technology. I do not have a definitive answer to that question. *Dr. Douglas M. Baird.*

Q. I must have surgery and I'm hypoglycemic. I'm not concerned about the procedure, but I am worried about the intravenous glucose. Is there anything else the doctors can give me instead?

A. Yes, there are other IV fluids that can be utilized in a hospital setting that will not affect your blood sugar. Ask your doctor. The stress of the surgery itself, however, may adversely affect your ability to manage your blood sugar. While this is a nuisance, it can be brought under control once you are back home. *Dr. Douglas M. Baird.*

Q. I have most of the symptoms of hypoglycemia, especially depression and mood swings. My doctor wants to put me on antidepressants. How can I convince him to take a glucose tolerance test first?

A. Depression and mood swings can certainly be a part of the symptom complex associated with hypoglycemia. They can also be symptoms of other disorders. The common work-up to begin to identify some of the underlying causes of these symptoms includes general chemistries, blood count, thyroid function testing and, if the symptoms warrant, glucose tolerance testing. If your doctor is unwilling to make the effort to eliminate the causes for your symptoms (for whatever reason), it may be time to consider seeking a second opinion. *Dr. Douglas M. Baird.*

Q.  Can hypoglycemia affect one's vision, and how?

A.  Blood sugar abnormalities can affect (and probably do) almost any tissue in one's body. The most dramatic effects are observed with brain function because the brain does not store readily available fuel. Other tissue areas are affected to a greater or lesser extent based on their individual susceptibility to blood sugar fluctuations as well as their fuel storage capabilities. The eye is an extension of the brain. It is a neutral tissue, does not store fuel and is susceptible to damage caused by reduced availability of fuel and/or oxygen. *Dr. Douglas M. Baird.*

Q.  I am 29 years old and have just been diagnosed as having hypoglycemia. I have been under a lot of stress and was wondering if this could have triggered the condition.

A.  To understand how stress can adversely affect this condition, a little physiology lesson might be in order. You cannot separate the psychological from the physical. You, as a total person, consist of both. When you suffer from stress (real or imagined), your physical body reacts with what is known as the "fight or flight" response. The adrenal glands secrete the catecholamines epinephrine and norepinephrine (adrenaline), which raise the blood glucose levels to prepare the body to fight or flee. Once that occurs, the pancreas begins to over-secrete insulin, and the blood glucose yo-yo begins. The drop in blood glucose is real! So, you need to be even more diligent with your diet during times of stress.

I also believe that once you understand how stress, like poor diet, can set off hypoglycemia, you will comprehend the need to control both. Also, the more overanxious you become about this condition, the more difficult it will be to get it under control. *Dr Lorna Walker.*

Q. What is your opinion about eating protein to manage low blood sugar?

A. Protein is not a "solution" to hypoglycemia. Protein can be used as a body fuel and is digested more slowly than carbohydrates and sugars. It is broken amino acids that can be turned into "fuel" later by the body if needed. Too much protein in the diet can lead to ketosis; too little can lead to protein starvation. The idea is to maintain a diet moderate in protein, low in carbohydrates (but not too low, as in the Atkins' diet) and devoid of simple sugars. This will help rest an overactive pancreas and help maintain steady blood glucose levels. *Dr. Lorna Walker.*

Q. I was recently diagnosed with hypoglycemia. My doctor prescribed a drug that has proved, in many cases, to reduce all signs of hypoglycemia. The drug is called Proglycem, which is not covered under my current insurance policy. I would like to know if you have any available information on this drug.

A. Proglycem (also known as Hyperstat) is a powerful drug used in the treatment of Hypertensive Emergency and "pathologic hypoglycemia due to insulinoma." An insulinoma is a tumor of the insulin-secreting cells of the pancreas. Functional hypoglycemia is not listed as one of the pharmaceutical indications for administration of this drug. In functional hypoglycemia, the insulin-secreting cells over secrete insulin in response to eating sugar and/or excessive refined carbohydrates. That is one reason why the fasting glucose levels of functional (reactive) hypoglycemia are usually within normal range. It is also why the condition is best treated with diet and lifestyle changes. I would surely consult a reputable endocrinologist before taking Proglycem for this condition. *Dr Lorna Walker.*

Q. I was diagnosed with hypoglycemia several years ago. I am currently suffering from a case of severe hives and am wondering if hypoglycemia has ever been known to cause this. Both my primary doctor and allergist don't seem to know what is causing this, so I am doing my own investigative work.

A. Hives indicate an allergic reaction to something. It is not hypoglycemia, although many hypoglycemics also suffer from allergies.

Although there is no scientific evidence to support it, I sometimes suspect that sub-clinical adrenal insufficiency may play a role in both disorders. The adrenal glands secrete glucocorticoids, which raise the blood glucose in times of stress or increased need. And hypoglycemics respond to rises in blood glucose with hyperinsulinism. Result: low blood glucose. The adrenals (along with the liver and other pancreatic hormones) must then secrete glucocorticoids to raise the blood sugar again. The cycle has begun.

Some adrenal hormones also serve to suppress the immune system and, in therapeutic doses, are used in the treatment of severe allergies and autoimmune disorders. If there are not enough of these types of hormones, the immune system may overreact to substances normally well tolerated, or "turn" on itself.

You will need to try to discover what your body is reacting to and remove it from your environment. *Dr Lorna Walker.*

Q. I've been having more trouble with my low blood sugar lately. I was wondering if there was a dietary way to get back to normal after a bout of very low blood sugar (near passing out). I know I need some juice at first, but what is the next best thing I should be eating after that and for the rest of the day?

A. Try not to respond to drops in blood sugar with sugar. It only continues the cycle of highs and lows. If you must drink some juice, dilute it with water, and then EAT something! A mixture of complex carbohydrates and protein usually works best. All the more reason to stick to your dietary regimen. The main purpose of the diet for hypoglycemia is to prevent drops in glucose, NOT to fix them after the fact. *Dr Lorna Walker.*

Q. My girlfriend has been diagnosed with Natal Hypoglycemia. From what I can make of the information available, low blood sugar can be caused by pregnancy and/or childbirth. Do you have any information on this condition?

A. Glucose Mismanagement Disorders are common to pregnancy. Both Gestational Diabetes and Gestational Hypoglycemia can occur. Many times the condition disappears after giving birth, but sometimes the stress of pregnancy is suspected of bringing out a condition that the woman is prone to anyway. In either case, the diet for hypoglycemia is compatible with pregnancy, as it is a healthy one. Be sure to have your girlfriend check with her doctor. *Dr Lorna Walker.*

Q. It is very rare that people talk about long-term, cumulative effects of hypoglycemic episodes. If one has a few dozen average-to-severe episodes per year of low blood sugar, what is the effect on various body functions? I have heard brain damage can result. Any suggestions?

A. The first organ affected by hypoglycemia is the brain, as its exclusive fuel is glucose. Unlike other organs, the brain cannot convert fats or protein to glucose. A few dozen short episodes a year have not proven to be detrimental. However, evidence is beginning to show that long-term, uncontrolled hypoglycemia could be a precursor to diabetes, the effects of which are well documented. All the more reason to stick to your dietary regimen. I say it repeatedly—the main purpose of the diet for hypoglycemia is to prevent drops in glucose, NOT to fix them after the fact. *Dr Lorna Walker.*

Q. Is there a way to do a glucose tolerance test at home?

A. Sorry, there is no way to do a glucose tolerance test at home. Many physicians familiar with this disorder often make the diagnosis by placing their patients on a hypoglycemic diet. If they improve, the diagnosis of hypoglycemia is made. Since the diet for hypoglycemia is a healthy one, I suggest you try eating as recommended and see if you feel better. *Dr Lorna Walker.*

Q. My son (18) has prostate cancer and was treated with chemotherapy. Now he has symptoms of hypoglycemia. Is there any connection?

A. Not necessarily. With the reference to the chemotherapy being the causative agent of the hypoglycemia, it would be extremely important to know which chemotherapy was used. Symptoms of hypoglycemia can occur that are not necessarily connected to the therapy given. Further, it would be important to determine if this is truly hypoglycemia or general immune suppression related to the chemotherapy. *Dr. Herbert Pardell.*

Q. I have hypoglycemia and chronic fatigue syndrome. Even though I'm on a strict hypoglycemia diet, I still can't seem to feel better. Is there anything I can do to speed the healing process?

A. Although you have not elucidated what you are doing at this time, I would assume that, under the circumstances, you are following protocols that include both diseases. The use of multiple antioxidants (which should of course include lipoic acid, selenium and chromium along with a strict diet) would help in this endeavor. Other parts of the protocol include a good exercise program along with proper rest. Each person is an individual, and the rate of healing depends on the general state of health and cannot be generalized for any one person. *Dr. Herbert Pardell.*

Q. I have hypoglycemia and hypothyroidism. Is this common?

A. The determination of commonality is very difficult because symptoms of both of these diseases seem to cross over and can be exhibited in either hypoglycemia or hypothyroidism. Decreased thyroid function will affect glucose metabolism and, in fact, will affect every part of the metabolic system, causing symptoms such as fatigue, sweating, weight gain, etc. Hypoglycemia can give you similar symptoms. At this time, I don't know of any studies that give an exact percentage of how many people have both entities. However, again the symptomatology of these diseases can be seen in either one. *Dr. Herbert Pardell.*

Q. I am hypoglycemic. I've heard and read that I should take chromium picolinate. How does it help, and how much should I take?

A. Chromium, whether it is given as chelate, picolinate or polynicotinate helps insulin work better to transport glucose to the cells. A big problem with insulin resistance is a deficiency of chromium and other trace elements. Without a mineral analysis, it is safe to take chromium as picolinate or chelate or polynicotinate at 200 to 400 mcg per day for adults. If you had a mineral analysis, we might recommend higher amounts. One word of caution: if you have high insulin levels and all your insulin is not sensitive, the chromium may initially activate it and you could experience worse blood sugar symptoms. If that happens, reduce or eliminate the chromium until you get further testing to see what you need. *Jay Foster, Nutritional Biochemist.*

Q. I am hypoglycemic and have been taking an herbal phen from the local health food store that has St. John's Wort and Ma Huang in it. Are there any health risks with this combination?

A. The Ma Huang may be dangerous. Many people using it report cardiac stress symptoms, including rapid heartbeat. The FDA is trying to get it banned. St. John's Wort is okay, but 50 mg. (a.m. & p.m.) of 5-HTP is better, although you cannot take either if you are on an SSRI drug like Paxil, Prozac or Zoloft. *Jay Foster, Nutritional Biochemist.*

Q. I've eliminated Aspartame and Nutrasweet. Can I have Splenda?

A. Research shows that the artificial sweetener Splenda, also known as sucralose, is a chlorinated sucrose derivative. I do not recommend it. For more information, use a search engine to look it up on the web. What you might try is Stevia. Stevia comes from a South American tree. It is natural, comes in pills, powder and liquid. I do not find the taste great, but other people find it very appealing. Also, research shows that it will do no harm. *Dr. Nancy Appleton.*

Q. How much sugar can a hypoglycemic ingest safely in one day?

A. I think a hypoglycemic should ingest very little sugar. This includes all forms of simple sugar such as sucrose, glucose, fructose, maltose, dextrose, honey, barley, malt, maple syrup, rice syrup, brown sugar, raw sugar, turbinado sugar, corn sweetener, corn syrup solids, liquid cane sugar, concentrated fruit juice, and fruit juice. The less, the better. There is plenty left to eat. If you eat fruit, eat it with protein and fat to control your blood sugar level. The fruits that have the least amount of sugar are melons and berries. *Dr. Nancy Appleton.*

Q. I am so confused. One book says I can eat whole wheat, and another book says I should avoid it. As a hypoglycemic trying to figure out what to eat, this is so confusing. What's correct?

A. Many people have made themselves allergic to wheat and dairy due to eating sugar with these products (cakes, cookies, pies, pastries, ice cream, cheesecake, yogurt, etc.). I do not think a hypoglycemic should eat any sugar, wheat, or dairy. The best foods to eat are whole foods, not processed foods like bread, boxed cereals, pasta, pizza, etc. *Dr. Nancy Appleton.*

Q. Is hypnosis recommended for hypoglycemia? I'm having a very difficult time with my diet. I can't seem to break my caffeine habits. I'm willing to try this but would this be the easy way out?

A. Although you could use hypnosis to try to gain control over longstanding habits, it is not necessarily the best treatment choice. The essential issue here is controlling cravings. The cravings you have are biologically driven. You may think they are a matter of will or psychological in some way, but when your blood sugar drops, you have little control over your food choices. Therefore, if you are following a proper hypoglycemic diet, the "cravings" should dissolve away. There are some food habits that are emotionally based. You will be able to see these once you have cut away the biologically driven ones. Examples include: eating comfort foods when upset or bored, or having a "relationship" with food in the place of the relationship you yearn for. If you feel you are eating from emotional need, a brief course of individual psychotherapy is a better treatment choice.

Regarding coffee, you must remember that caffeine is a drug from which you must withdraw slowly. Go slowly and replace it with a healthy alternative. Don't overlook how powerful this morning ritual is and brew herbal/green tea instead of coffee if that is your replacement. *Dr. Nancy Scheinman.*

Q. I've just been diagnosed as having hypoglycemia after years of being told that my symptoms "were all in my head." I'm not only having a hard time with my diet but with my emotions. I am so a angry at all the doctors, my family included, who never really believed that this is a tried and true condition. I'm working on my diet but how can I get past my anger?

A. The only reason why the people in your past labeled your hypoglycemia as "all in your head." was because they had no understanding of what was actually taking place. Can you really be angry at someone because they have never been exposed to something? Or because, generally, our knowledge of the disease is in a developmental state? They weren't making a value judgement about you: they were merely reaching for the only reason they could find. I notice that the solution to a problem does not appear until a person is truly ready to see it and confront it. That is, ask yourself these questions: "Was I really ready to deal with this back then? How have I grown from the difficulty of living with this? Who am I as a result of this?"

Anger is a complex emotion. While it may be destructive, it may also be motivating and empowering. The key is to change the energy of the anger into a positive force. Interestingly, if you do not, and you remain stuck in the anger, it may actually interfere with your sugar. By remaining angry, you may create blood sugar instability. Therefore, via another route, you will allow these individuals to continue to block your healing. *Dr. Nancy Scheinman.*

Q. My nine year old daughter was diagnosed as having hypoglycemia. I changed her diet, which consisted of a large amount of sugar and fruit juices. She was doing quite well until I started giving her a vitamin/mineral supplement. I thought this was a good idea. Why does she seem worse since I added this chewable?

A. I just addressed this problem in a recent article that I wrote in *the Journal of Longevity.* You child may be allergic to some of the additives in the supplement. Our research has shown that about seven percent of the population has chemical sensitivities to a variety of things like synthetic food colors, food dyes, binders, and fillers. (Incidentally, many food dyes, binders, and emulsifiers have been linked to Attention Deficit Hyperactivity Disorder (ADHD) and hyperactivity alone.) For example, although kids prefer chewable vitamin supplements, all chewables contain the exact same chemicals, which we know promote hyperactivity. Unfortunately, there's no known technology for creating a chewable without using these chemicals. For those kids who are chemically sensitive, hypoallergenic nutritional supplements are the answer. *Dr. Stephen J. Schoenthaler.*

# ⋙Chapter 17

RECOMMENDED
FOODS/MENUS

## *Recommended Foods*

N ote: The following list of recommended foods and menus is just a guideline. You must remember that everyone's body chemistry is different, therefore, adjustments must be made to meet individual needs. Size of portions depend on weight and symptoms. READ the chapter on INDIVIDUALIZING YOUR DIET before incorporating the menus into your diet program.

Meats:     All kinds of fresh meats—veal, lamb, lean beef, pork (if no nitrates).

Poultry:   Without skin—chicken, turkey, Cornish hens, duck, pheasant.

Fish:      Flounder, turbot, sole, halibut, grouper, cod, haddock, salmon, red snapper, scallops, tuna, shrimp, lobster, crab.

Dairy:     Whole milk, skim milk, cheeses (farmer, cottage, ricotta, mozzarella), eggs, butter and yogurt.

165

Grains: 100 percent whole wheat bread, brown rice, millet, oatmeal, buckwheat, oats, whole wheat pasta and noodles.

Nuts & Seeds: Almonds, cashews, walnuts, pecans, chestnuts, sunflower seeds, pumpkin seeds.

Vegetables: Artichokes, asparagus, avocado, beans, beets, broccoli, brussels sprouts, cabbage, carrots, cauliflower, celery, chives, collard greens, corn, cucumber, eggplant, endive, garlic, kale, lettuce, mushrooms, mustard greens, okra, onion, parsley, peas, peppers, potatoes, pumpkin, radish, rhubarb, spinach, sprouts, tomatoes, zucchini, and yams.

Beverages: Water, vegetable juice, herbal tea, seltzer, clear-broth. Occasionally, decaffeinated coffee or weak tea.

Fruits: Avocado, strawberries, apples, peaches, pears, oranges, watermelon, tangerines, berries, plums, grapefruit, honeydew.

## *Foods to Avoid*

Desserts: Anything containing white sugar, such as, candy, cakes, pastries, custard, jello, icecream, sherbet, pudding, cookies, breakfast cereals, and commercially baked breads. Avoid honey and other forms of sugar, such as brown, raw, and turbinado.

Grains: Anything containing white flour, such as packaged breakfast cereals, gravies, white rice, refined corn meal, white spaghetti, macaroni, noodles and refined bakery goods.

Meats: Lunch meats, bacon, sausage, processed meats (most contain corn sugar), meat or meat products with artificial colors, flavorings or preservatives.

Beverages: Alcohol, caffeine, all sugared soft drinks, and fruit juices.

Fruits: Dried fruits (figs, dates, raisins). Fruit juices can be tolerated at times if diluted. Avoid EXCESSIVE amounts of fresh fruit.

*Note: Tobacco should be avoided entirely.*

## *Suggested List of Snacks*

FRESH VEGETABLES: tomato wedges, sliced cucumbers, carrot, celery sticks, radish flowers, sliced summer squash, zucchini, cauliflower, broccoli flowerettes (steamed) mushrooms, and pepper rings.

FRESH FRUITS: apple wedges, orange slices, cantaloupe, watermelon, and strawberries (in moderation)

COTTAGE CHEESE
HARD BOILED EGG
YOGURT
GRANOLA SEEDS (sesame, sunflower, pumpkin)
NUTS (almonds, cashews, pecans, walnuts)
POPCORN
COLD CHICKEN, TURKEY, ROAST BEEF
CHEESE SLICES
WHOLE GRAIN BREAD (with nut butter)
RICE CRACKERS (with natural peanut butter, tuna fish or cheese)
RICE WAFERS (with natural peanut butter, tuna fish or cheese)
WHOLE WHEAT PRETZELS
APPLESAUCE (no sugar)
CELERY STICKS (stuffed with peanut butter, tuna fish or cheese)
BAKED POTATO (with steamed vegetables)

## *Suggested Breakfast*

1/2 cup of oatmeal
1 poached egg
1/2 grapefruit
Beverage


1 egg omelet with green peppers, onions or mushrooms
1 slice whole wheat bread or rice cake
1 orange
Beverage


1/2 cup of cream of rice (millet, grits, dry rolled oats)
Cheese omelet
1 cup strawberries
Beverage


1 - 2 slices of whole grain bread
1 cup cottage cheese
Beverage

## *Suggested Lunches & Dinners*

Chef salad (egg, turkey, chicken, lettuce, carrots, etc.), with
oil and vinegar dressing
1 slice whole wheat bread or rice cake
Beverage

Soup (bean, lentil, chicken or beef)
Small tossed salad
1 slice whole wheat bread
Beverage

4 - 6 oz. broiled shrimp (or fish of any kind)
Green beans with almonds (or mushrooms)
Small tossed salad
Beverage

4 - 6 oz. chicken (one leg, thigh or breast)
1 small potato
Broccoli
Small tossed salad
Beverage

Broiled lamb chop
Brown rice
Brussels sprouts
Small tossed salad
Beverage

# Health Emergency Card

This card was custom-designed with the hypoglycemic in mind. It should be kept close to your side at all times! Feel secure knowing that your diagnosis, allergies, medications, and physician are listed on this card in the event of an emergency. Enjoy peace of mind knowing that this card will contain vital information that could *save your life!*

To order your Health Emergency Card, please mail in a check for $12.00 plus postage:

| | |
|---|---|
| First Class: | $2.50 |
| Priory Mail: | $4.50 |
| Out of the U.S.: | $8.50. |

Please include a picture of the card holder (no larger that 5"x7") and your check or Money Order to:

**The Hypoglycemia Support Foundation, Inc.**
**P.O. Box 451778**
**Sunrise, Fl 33345**
Please allow 2-4 weeks delivery

To use your credit card, please visit our website:
**www.hypoglycemia.org**

# Health Emergency Card
## Order Form

First Name:
Last Name:

Address:
City:          State:          Zip:
Country:

Email:
Date of Birth:
Sex:  Male   Female
Home phone:    Work Phone:
Emergency Contact:    Emergency Phone:
Diagnosis:
Allergies:
Medication:
Physician Name:
Physician's Phone:

## HEALTH EMERGENCY CARD

**Roberta Ruggiero**
P.O. Box 451778
**Sunrise, FL 33322**

| Home Phone | Work Phone | D.O.B. | Sex |
|---|---|---|---|
|  |  |  | F |

| Emergency Contact | Emergency Number |
|---|---|
| Anthony Ruggiero |  |

| | |
|---|---|
| Diagnosis | Hypoglycemia |
| Allergies | Penicillin |
| Medication | Cytomel |
| Physician | Dr. Herbert Pardell |

**The Hypoglycemia Support Foundation, Inc.**

172

# Hypoglycemia Quiz: Diet/Symptom Diary

## HYPOGLYCEMIA: DO YOU HAVE IT?

I n the space provided below, please mark ( 1 ) if you have this condition mildly, (2) if moderate, and (3) if severe. If you do not have the condition, leave it blank. The accuracy of this questionnaire depends upon complete honesty and serious objective thought in answering the questions. (Many of these symptoms may relate to other health problems).

1____Abnormal craving for sweets

2____Afternoon headaches

3____Allergies: tendency to asthma, hay fever, skin rash, etc.

4____Awaken after a few hours sleep/difficulty getting back to sleep

5____Aware of breathing heavily

6____Bad dreams

7____Blurred vision

8____Brown spots or bronzing of skin

9____"Butterfly stomach," cramps

10____Difficulty making decisions

11____Need coffee/caffeine to start morning

12____unable to work under pressure

13____Chronic fatigue

14____Chronic nervous exhaustion

15____Convulsions

16____Crave candy or coffee in afternoons

17____Cry easily for no apparent reason

18____Depressed

19____Dizziness, giddiness or light-headedness

20____Drink more than three cups of coffee or cola a day

21____Get hungry or feel faint unless you eat frequently

22____Eat when nervous

23____Feel faint if meal is delayed

24____Fatigue relieved by eating

25____Fearful

26____Get "shaky" if hungry

27____Hallucinations

28____Hand tremor (or trembles)

29____Heart palpitations if meals are missed or delayed

30____Highly emotional

31____Nibble between meals because of hunger

32____Insomnia

33____Inward trembling

34____Irritable before meals

35____Lack of energy

36____Moods of depression, "blues" or melancholy

37____Poor memory or ability to concentrate
38____Reduced initiative
39____Sleepy after meals
40____Drowsy during the day
41____Weakness, dizziness
42____Worrier, feel insecure
43____Symptoms of hypoglycemia appear before eating
44____Total Score.

Add the total of all answers. A total score of less than (20) twenty is within normal limits. A higher score is evidence of probable adrenal insufficiency and/or deranged carbohydrate metabolism (Hypoglycemia), and would indicate further testing.

# ᴤAppendix A

*Blood Sugar Blues,* Miryam Ehrlich Williamson, Walker & Company, New York 2001.

*Body, Mind and Sugar*, by E.M. Abrahamson, M.D. and A.W. Pezet. New York, Avon Books, 1977.

*Carlton Fredericks' New Low Blood Sugar and You*, by Dr.Carlton Fredericks. NewYork, Perigee Books, 1985.

*Dr. Atkins' New Diet Revolution* by Robert C. Atkins, M.D., M. Evans, 1992.

*Food, Mind and Mood*, by David Sheinkin, M.D., Michael Schacter, M.D., and Richard Hutton. New York, Warner Books, Inc., 1979.

*Fighting Depression*, by Harvey Ross, M.D., New York, Larchmont Books, 1975.

*Get the Sugar Out* by Ann Louise Gittleman, M.S.,
New York: Crown trade Paperbacks, 1996.

*The Hidden Menace of Low Blood Sugar*, by Clement G.
Martin. New York, Arco Publishing Co., 1976.

*Hypoglycemia: A Better Approach*, by Paavo Airola, Ph.D.
Phoenix, Health Plus Publishers, 1977.

*Is Low Blood Sugar Making You a Nutritional Cripple?* by
Ruth Adams and Frank Murray. New York, Larchmont
Press, 1970.

*Lick The Sugar Habit*, by Nancy Appleton, Ph.D. New York,
Warner Books, Inc., 1986.

*Low Blood Sugar Handbook*, by Ed and Patricia Krimmel.
Bryn Mawr, PA, Franklin Publishers, 1984.

*Low Blood Sugar*; What it Is and How to Cure It, by Peter
J. Steincrohn, M.D., Chicago, Ill., Contemporary Books,
Inc.,1972.

*Nutraerobics*, by Dr. Jeffrey Bland, New York, Harper and
Row, 1983.

*Psychodietetics*, by Emanuel Cheraskin, M.D., D.M.D., William Ringsdorf, Jr., D.M.D. with Arline Brecher. New York, Bantam Books, 1978.

*Seven Weeks to Sobriety; The Proven Program to Fight Alcoholism Through Nutrition* by Joan Mathews Larson, Ph. D., Ballantine publishing Group, 1997.

*Sugar and Your Health*, by Ray C. Wunderlich, Jr., M.D. St. Petersburg, FL, Good Health Publications, Johnny Reed, Inc., 1982.

*Sugar Blues*, by William Dufty. New York, Warner Books, Inc., 1975.
*Sugar Isn't Always Sweet*, by Maura (Jinny) Zack and Wilbur D. Currier, M.D. Brea, CA, Uplift Books, 1983.

*Sweet and Dangerous*, by John Yudkin, M.D. New York, Bantam Books, 1972.

*The Sugar Addict's Total Recovery Program,* by kathleen Des Maisons, Ph.D., Ballantine Publishing Group.

## *Cookbooks for the Hypoglycemic*

*The Allergy Cookbook*, by Ruth R. Shattuck. NewYork, A
   Plume Book, 1984.

*Cooking Naturally For Pleasure and Health*, by Gail C.
   Watson. Davie, FL, Falkynor Books, 1983.

*Foods For Healthy Kids*, by Dr. Lendon Smith. New York,
   Berkeley Books, 1981.

*Hypoglycemia Control Cookery*, by Dorothy Revell. New
   York, Berkeley Books, 1973.

*The Low Blood Sugar Cookbook*, by Francyne Davis.   New
   York, Bantam Books, 1985.

*Dr. Lendon Smith's Diet Plan For Teenagers*, by Lendon
   Smith, M.D. NewYork, McGraw-Hill, 1986.
*Step-By-Step To Natural Food*, by Diane Campbell.
   Clearwater, FL, CC Publishers, 1979.

*Sugar Free. . .That's Me*, by Judith S. Majors. New York,
   Ballantine Books, 1978.

*The Low Blood Sugar Cookbook*, by Ed and Patricia
   Krimmel, Bryn Mawr, PA, Franklin Publishers, 1984.

## *Exercise Books for the Hypoglycemic*

*Aerobics,* by Kenneth H. Cooper, M.D., NewYork, Bantam, 1972.

*Aerobics For Women,* by Kenneth H. Cooper, M.D., New York, Bantam Books, 1973.

*The Aerobics Program For Total Well-Being,* by Kenneth H. Cooper, M.D., New York, Bantam, 1983.

*The Complete Book of Exercisewalking,* by Gary D. Yanker. Contemporary Books, Inc., 1983.

*Fit or Fat? by Covert Bailey. Boston,* Houghton Mifflin Company, 1977.

*Gary Yanker's Sportwalking,* by Gary Yanker, New York Contemporary Books, 1987.

## *Books to Help Develop a Positive Attitude*

*Anatomy of An Illness,* by Norman Cousins, New York, W.W. Norton & Co., 1979.

*Bus 9 To Paradise, by Leo Buscaglia,* New York, Fawcett, 1987.

*Enthusiasm Makes the Difference*, by Norman Vincent Peale, NewYork, Fawcett, 1987.

*Gifts Form Eykis*, by Dr. Wayne Dyer, New York, Pocket Books, 1983.

*Goodbye to Guilt*, by Gerald G. Jampolsky, M.D., New York, Bantam Books, Inc., 1985.

*The Healing Heart*, by Norman Cousins, New York, Avon Books, 1983.

*Love,* by Leo Buscaglia, New York, Fawcett Crest Books, 1972.
*Loving Each Other*, by Leo Buscaglia, NewYork, Fawcett Columbine, 1984.

*Personhood*, by Leo Buscaglia, New York, Fawcett Columbine, 1978.

*The Power of Positive Thinking*, by Norman Vincent Peale, NewYork, Prentice-Hall, Inc., 1952.

*Pulling Your Own Strings*, by Dr. Wayne Dyer, New York, Thomas Y. Crowell Co., 1978.

*The Road Less Traveled*, by M. Scott Peck, M.D., New
York, Simon and Schuster, 1978.

*Tough Times Never Last*, But Tough People Do!, by Robert
H. Schuller, NewYork, Bantam Books, 1983.

*The Seat of the Soul* by Gary Zukav, Simon & Shuster, 1990.

*The Sky's The Limit*, by Dr. Wayne Dyer, New York,
Simon and Schuster, 1980.

*Teach Only Love: The Seven Principles of Attitudinal Healing*,
by Gerald G. Jampolsky, M.D., New York, Bantam, 1983.

*When Bad Things Happen to Good People*, by Harold S.
Kushner, New York, Avon Books, 1981.

*Your Erroneous Zones*, by Dr. Wayne Dyer, New York,
Funk & Wagnalls, 1976.

§

## *Books on the Correlation Between Hypoglycemia & Learning Disabilities, Juvenile Delinquency, Mental Illness, Alcoholism and Candida Albicans*

*Allergies and the Hyperactive Child,* by Doris J. Rapp, M.D. NewYork, Simon & Schuster, 1979.

*Brain Allergies,* by William H. Philpott, M.D. and Dwight K. Kalita, Ph.D. New Canaan, CT, 1980.

*Chocolate to Morphine,* by Andrew Weil, M.D., and Winifred Rosen. Boston, Houghton Mifflin, 1968.

*Diet, Crime and Delinquency,* by Alexander Schauss, Ph.D. Berkeley, CA, Parker House, 1981.

*Eating Right To Live Sober,* by L. Ann Mueller, M.D., and Katherine Ketchum, NewYork, NAL, 1986.

*Fighting Depression,* by Harvey Ross, M.D., New York, Larchmont Books, 1975.

*Food, Teens and Behavior,* by Barbara Reed Stitt,Ph.D. Manitowoc, WI, Natural Press, 1983.

*Hypoglycemia: A Better Approach,* by Paavo Airola, Ph.D. Phoenix, Health Plus Publishers, 1977.

*Mind, Mood and Medicine: A Guide To The New Biopsychiatry,* by Paul H. Wender, M.D. and Donald F. Klein, M.D., NewYork, NAL, 1982.

*Psychodietetics,* by E. Cheraskin, M.D., D.M.D., William Ringsdorf Jr., D.M.D. with Arline Brecher. NewYork, Bantam Books, 1978.

*Sugar and Your Health,* by Ray C. Wunderlich, Jr., M.D. St. Petersburg, FL Good Health Publications, 1982.

*The Yeast Connection,* by William G. Crook, M.D., Jackson, Tenn., Professional Books, 1983.

*The Yeast Syndrome,* by John Parks Trowbridge, M.D. and Morton Walker, D.P.M., 1986.

§

# ᴁ(Appendix B

Hypoglycemia Support Foundation, Inc.,
Frederick Fell Publishers, Inc.,
2131 Hollywood Blvd. Suite 305
Hollywood, FL 33020.

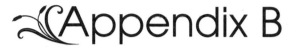

Hypoglycemia Association, Inc.
18008 New Hampshire Ave
Box 165
Ashton, Maryland 20861-0165
Recorded Message
Phone:    (202) 544-4044

International Academy of Preventive Medicine,
34 Corporate Woods, Suite 469,
10950 Grandview,
Overland Park, KS 66210.

International Academy of Applied Nutrition,
P.O. Box 386
La Habra, CA 90631.

The Price-Pottenger Nutrition Foundation
P.O. Box 2614
La Mesa, California 91943-2614
Phone:    (619) 574-7763
E-mail:    www.Price-Pottinger.org

American Holistic Medical Association
12101 Menaul Boulevard NE
Mc Lean, Virginia 22101
Phone:      (703) 556-9245
E-mail:    www.holisticmedicine.org

American Chiropractic Association,
1701 Clarendon Blvd., Arlington, VA 22209.
American Academy of Osteopathy
3500 DePauw Boulevard Suite 1080
Indianapolis, Indiana 46268
Phone:    (317) 879-1881
Fax:       (317) 879-0563
E-mail:    www.academyofosteopathy.org

American College for Advancement in Medicine
23121 Verdugo Drive
Suite 202
Laguna, California 92653
Phone:    1-800-532-3688
E-mail:    ACAM.org

The Life Extension Foundation
1100 W. Commercial Boulevard
Fort Lauderdale, Florida 33309
Phone:   (954) 766-8433 or 1-800-226-2370
E-mail:   www.LifeExtension.com

Well Mind Association of Greater Washington
18606 New Hampshire Avenue
Ashton, Maryland 20861-9789
Phone:   (301) 774-6617
Fax:      (301) 774-0536

§

189

# Appendix C

## BIBLIOGRAPHY

Abrahamson, E.M., M.D., and Pezet, A.W.  Body, Mind and
 Sugar. NewYork, Avon Books, 1977.

Adams, Ruth, and Murray, Frank.  Is Low Blood Sugar
 Making You a Nutritional Cripple? New York,
 Larchmont Press, 1970.

Airola, Paavo, Ph.D.  Hypoglycemia: A Better Approach.
 Phoenix, Health Plus Publishers, 1977.

Anderson, Linnea, M.P.H., Dibble, Marjorie V., M.S., R.D.,
 Turkki, Pirkko R., Ph.D., R.D., Mitchell, Helen S.,
 Ph.D., Sc.D., Rynbergen, HenderikaJ., M.S.
 Nutrition in Health and Disease, 17th Edition.
 Philadelphia, J.B. Lippincott Company.

Appleton, Nancy, Ph.D.  Lick the Sugar Habit. New York,
 Warner Books, Inc. 1986.

Atkinson, Holly, M.D. Women and Fatigue.  NewYork,
 G.P. Putnam's Sons, 1985.

Bailey, Covert. Fit or Fat? Boston, Houghton Mifflin Company, 1977.

Bennion, Lynn J., M.D. Hypoglycemia: Fact or Fad? New York, Crown Publishers, Inc. 1983.

Bland, Jeffery, Ph.D. Your Health Under Siege. Vermont, The Stephen Greene Press, 1981.

Brennan, Dr. R.O. Nutrigenetics. NewYork, M. Evans and Company, 1975.

Budd, Martin L., N.D., D.O., Lic.Ac. Low Blood Sugar. New York, Sterling Publishing Co., Inc. 1981.

Cheraskin, E., M.D., D.M.D., William Ringsdorf, Jr., D.M.D. and .W. Clark, D.D.S., Diet and Disease. Connecticut, Keats Publishing, Inc. 1986.

Cheraskin E., M.D., D.M.D., William Ringsdorf, Jr., D.M.D., with Arline Brecher. Phychodietetics. New York, Bantam Books, 1978.

Cheraskin, E., M.D., D.M.D., William Ringsdorf, Jr., D.M.D., and Emily L. Sisley, Ph.D. The Vitamin C Connection. NewYork, Harper & Row Publishers, Inc., 1983.

Crook, William G., M.D.  The Yeast Connection. Tennessee, Professional Books, 1983.

Dufty, William. Sugar Blues.  New York, Warner Books, Inc., 1975.

Fredericks, Carlton, Ph.D.  Carlton Fredericks' New Low Blood Sugar and You. New York, Perigee Books, 1985.

Fredericks, Carlton, Ph.D.  Psycho-Nutrition. NewYork, Grosset & Dunlap, 1976.

Krimmel, Patricia and Edward.  The Low Blood Sugar Handbook. Bryn Mawr, PA, Franklin Publishers, 1984.

Lorenzani, Shirley, Ph.D.  Candida; A Twentieth Century Disease. New Canaan, CT, Keats Publishing, Inc., 1986.

Martin, Clement G.  Low Blood Sugar; The Hidden Menace of Hypoglycemia. New York, Arco Publishing Co., 1976.

The Merck Manual of Diagnosis and Therapy, Twelfth Edition. Rahway, NJ, Merck Sharp & Dohme Research Laboratories, Division of Merck & Co., Inc.

Milam, James R. and Katherine Ketcham, Under the Influence, New York, Bantam Books, 1981.

Nutrition and Mental Health. Hearing before the Select
Committee on Nutrition and Human Needs of the
United States Senate. California, Parker House, 1977.

Page, Melvin E., D.D.S., and H. Leon Abrams, Jr. Your
Body is Your Best Doctor. New Canaan, CT, Keats
Publishing, 1972.

Passwater, Richard A. Supernutrition. New York, Pocket
Books, 1975.

Pritikin, Nathan, with Patrick M. McGrady, Jr. The Pritikin
Program for Diet and Exercise. New York, Grosset &
Dunlap, 1979.

Rapp, Doris, J., M.D. Allergies and the Hyperactive Child.
NewYork,Simon&Schuster,1979.

Reed, Barbara. Foods,Teens and Behavior. Manitowoc,Wi,
Natural Press, 1983.
Ross, Harvey, M.D. Fighting Depression. NewYork,
Larchmont Books, 1975.

Schauss, Alexander,Diet, Crime and Delinquency. Berkeley,
CA, Parker House, 1981.

Saunders, Jeraldine, and Ross, Harvey, M.D. Hypoglycemia:

The Disease Your Doctor Won't Treat, New
York Pinnacle Press, 1980.

Smith, Lendon, M.D.  Feed Yourself Right. New York,
McGraw-Hill, 1983.

Smith, Lendon, M.D.  Foods For Healthy Kids. New York,
Berkeley Books, 1981.

Truss, C. Orion, M.D.  The Missing Diagnosis. Birmingham,
The Missing Diagnosis, Inc., 1983.

Yudkin, John M.D.  Sweet and Dangerous. New York,
Bantam Books, 1972.

Weil, Andrew, M.D., and Rosen, Winifred.  Chocolate to
Morphine. Boston, Houghton Mifflin Co., 1983.

Weller, Charles.  How To Live With Hypoglycemia. New
York, Doubleday, 1968.

Wunderlich, Jr., Ray C., M.D.  Sugar and Your Health. St
Petersburg, FL, Good Health Publications, Johnny
Reed, Inc., 1982.

Zack, Maura and Currier, Wilbur D., M.D. Sugar Isn't Always
Sweet. Brea, CA, Uplift Books, 1983.

# Index

§

**P**
pancreas, 31, 55-56, 166-167, 175, 180-182
phobias, 56
Pardell, Dr. Herbert, 174, 186-187
positive attitude, 50, 62 119,128
pregnancy, 33, 153, 184
**R**
Rapp, Dr. Doris, 140
Ross, Dr. Harvey, 60, 111, 155
**S**
Saunders, Jeraldine, 164
schizophrenia, 77, 92
sleeping in class, 144
snacks, 73-74, 76, 79, 142, 150, 196
Schoenthaler, Dr. Stephen J, 52, 174, 192
Smith, Dr. Lenden, 140
splenda, 188
St. John's Wort, 188
Stein, Carolyn, 125
stevia, 188
stress, 43, 55, 57, 80, 90, 98-99, 101, 105, 115, 122, 128,
        133-135, 140, 143, 175-176, 179-181, 183-184, 188
Students Against Drunk Drivers (SADD), 154
sucralose, 188
sudden hunger, 40, 56
support groups, 116, 120, 150
surgery, 179
**T**
teenagers, 137, 139, 144, 173
therapy, benefits of, 111
tobacco, 55, 57, 69, 71-72, 76, 79, 98, 144, 146, 156, 160, 170
**V**
Valium, 60, 67, 120
vision, 46, 56, 170, 180, 201
vitamins, 26, 49-50, 76, 95-102, 104, 111, 128, 142, 149, 157,
        160, 168, 177, 192
**W**
Walker, Dr. Lorna, 52, 166, 173, 181-185
walking, 104-106
Williams, Dr. David, 155

The Hypoglycemia Research Foundation, Inc.
was founded
on June 6, 1980
but was renamed
The Hypoglycemia Support Foundation, Inc.
on December 13, 1991.